MW01181206

This book belongs to:

DATE	/ /	DAY	Mon	Tue	Wed	Thu	Fri	Sat	Sun

Time

Begin		End		Duration	
Begin		End		Duration	
Begin		End		Duration	

Location

- ☐ Tension
- ☐ Neck
- ☐ Migraine
- ☐ Cluster
- ☐ GCA
- ☐ Sinus

Severity

MILD ① ② ③ ④ ⑤ ⑥ ⑦ ⑧ ⑨ ⑩ SEVERE

Triggers

◯ Coffee	◯ Bright light	◯ Eye strain	◯ Commute
◯ Alcohol	◯ Stress	◯ Pc/Tv screen	◯ Pms
◯ Medication	◯ Anxiety	◯ Hunger	◯ Others
◯ Food	◯ Reading	◯ Insomnia	◯
◯ Weather	◯ Noise	◯ Smell	◯
◯ Allergies	◯ Motion	◯ Sickness	◯

RELIEF MEASURES

Medication	
Water	
Sleep	
Exercise	
Other	

Notes

DATE	/ /	DAY	Mon	Tue	Wed	Thu	Fri	Sat	Sun

Time

Begin		End		Duration	
Begin		End		Duration	
Begin		End		Duration	

Location

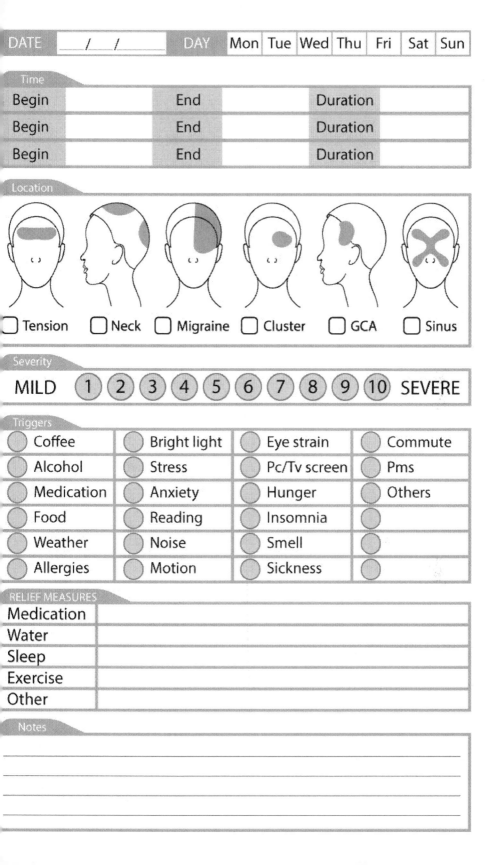

- ☐ Tension
- ☐ Neck
- ☐ Migraine
- ☐ Cluster
- ☐ GCA
- ☐ Sinus

Severity

MILD (1) (2) (3) (4) (5) (6) (7) (8) (9) (10) SEVERE

Triggers

◯ Coffee	◯ Bright light	◯ Eye strain	◯ Commute
◯ Alcohol	◯ Stress	◯ Pc/Tv screen	◯ Pms
◯ Medication	◯ Anxiety	◯ Hunger	◯ Others
◯ Food	◯ Reading	◯ Insomnia	◯
◯ Weather	◯ Noise	◯ Smell	◯
◯ Allergies	◯ Motion	◯ Sickness	◯

RELIEF MEASURES

Medication	
Water	
Sleep	
Exercise	
Other	

Notes

DATE	___/___/___	DAY	Mon	Tue	Wed	Thu	Fri	Sat	Sun

Begin		End		Duration	
Begin		End		Duration	
Begin		End		Duration	

Location

- ☐ Tension
- ☐ Neck
- ☐ Migraine
- ☐ Cluster
- ☐ GCA
- ☐ Sinus

Severity

MILD ①②③④⑤⑥⑦⑧⑨⑩ SEVERE

Triggers

Coffee	Bright light	Eye strain	Commute
Alcohol	Stress	Pc/Tv screen	Pms
Medication	Anxiety	Hunger	Others
Food	Reading	Insomnia	
Weather	Noise	Smell	
Allergies	Motion	Sickness	

RELIEF MEASURES

Medication	
Water	
Sleep	
Exercise	
Other	

Notes

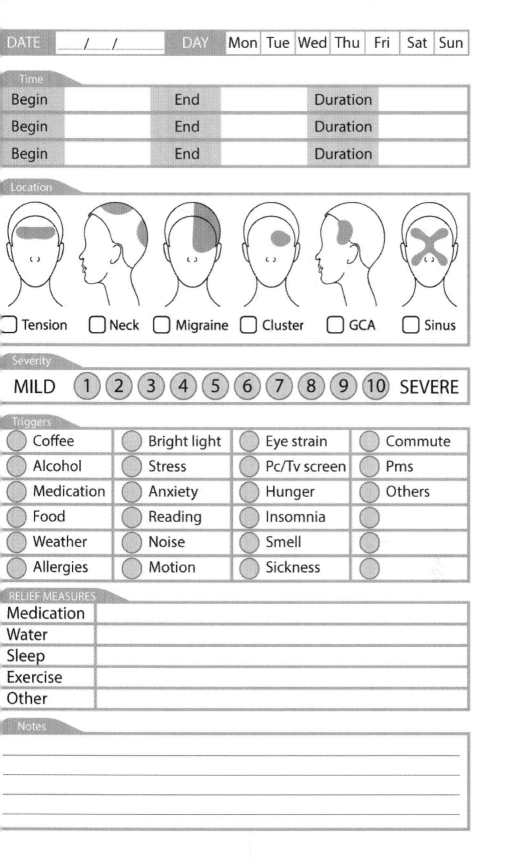

| DATE | / / | | DAY | Mon | Tue | Wed | Thu | Fri | Sat | Sun |

Time

Begin		End		Duration	
Begin		End		Duration	
Begin		End		Duration	

Location

☐ Tension ☐ Neck ☐ Migraine ☐ Cluster ☐ GCA ☐ Sinus

Severity

MILD ① ② ③ ④ ⑤ ⑥ ⑦ ⑧ ⑨ ⑩ SEVERE

Triggers

○ Coffee	○ Bright light	○ Eye strain	○ Commute
○ Alcohol	○ Stress	○ Pc/Tv screen	○ Pms
○ Medication	○ Anxiety	○ Hunger	○ Others
○ Food	○ Reading	○ Insomnia	○
○ Weather	○ Noise	○ Smell	○
○ Allergies	○ Motion	○ Sickness	○

RELIEF MEASURES

Medication	
Water	
Sleep	
Exercise	
Other	

Notes

DATE	/ /	DAY	Mon	Tue	Wed	Thu	Fri	Sat	Sun

Time

Begin		End		Duration	
Begin		End		Duration	
Begin		End		Duration	

Location

☐ Tension ☐ Neck ☐ Migraine ☐ Cluster ☐ GCA ☐ Sinus

Severity

MILD ① ② ③ ④ ⑤ ⑥ ⑦ ⑧ ⑨ ⑩ SEVERE

Triggers

○ Coffee	○ Bright light	○ Eye strain	○ Commute
○ Alcohol	○ Stress	○ Pc/Tv screen	○ Pms
○ Medication	○ Anxiety	○ Hunger	○ Others
○ Food	○ Reading	○ Insomnia	○
○ Weather	○ Noise	○ Smell	○
○ Allergies	○ Motion	○ Sickness	○

RELIEF MEASURES

Medication	
Water	
Sleep	
Exercise	
Other	

Notes

DATE	/ /	DAY	Mon	Tue	Wed	Thu	Fri	Sat	Sun

Time

Begin		End		Duration	
Begin		End		Duration	
Begin		End		Duration	

Location

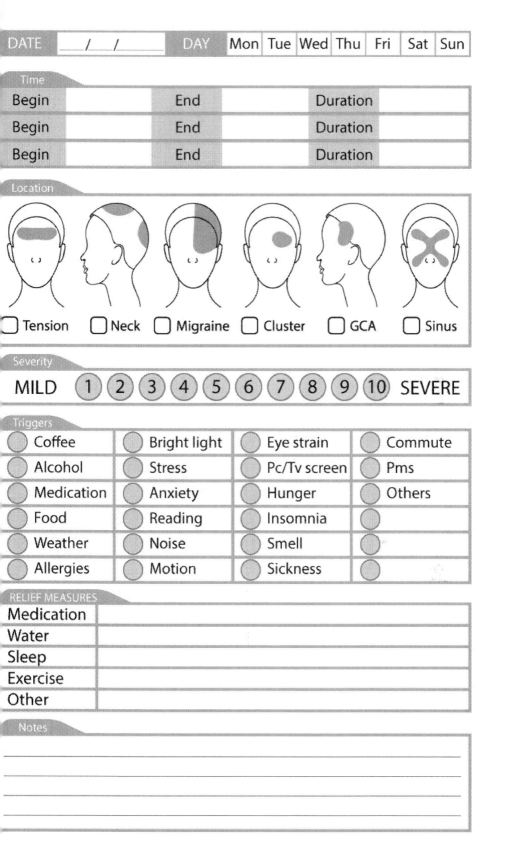

☐ Tension ☐ Neck ☐ Migraine ☐ Cluster ☐ GCA ☐ Sinus

Severity

MILD (1) (2) (3) (4) (5) (6) (7) (8) (9) (10) SEVERE

Triggers

◯ Coffee	◯ Bright light	◯ Eye strain	◯ Commute
◯ Alcohol	◯ Stress	◯ Pc/Tv screen	◯ Pms
◯ Medication	◯ Anxiety	◯ Hunger	◯ Others
◯ Food	◯ Reading	◯ Insomnia	◯
◯ Weather	◯ Noise	◯ Smell	◯
◯ Allergies	◯ Motion	◯ Sickness	◯

RELIEF MEASURES

Medication	
Water	
Sleep	
Exercise	
Other	

Notes

DATE	/ /	DAY	Mon	Tue	Wed	Thu	Fri	Sat	Sun

Time

Begin		End		Duration	
Begin		End		Duration	
Begin		End		Duration	

Location

☐ Tension   ☐ Neck   ☐ Migraine   ☐ Cluster   ☐ GCA   ☐ Sinus

Severity

MILD (1) (2) (3) (4) (5) (6) (7) (8) (9) (10) SEVERE

Triggers

○ Coffee	○ Bright light	○ Eye strain	○ Commute
○ Alcohol	○ Stress	○ Pc/Tv screen	○ Pms
○ Medication	○ Anxiety	○ Hunger	○ Others
○ Food	○ Reading	○ Insomnia	○
○ Weather	○ Noise	○ Smell	○
○ Allergies	○ Motion	○ Sickness	○

RELIEF MEASURES

Medication	
Water	
Sleep	
Exercise	
Other	

Notes

_____
_____
_____
_____

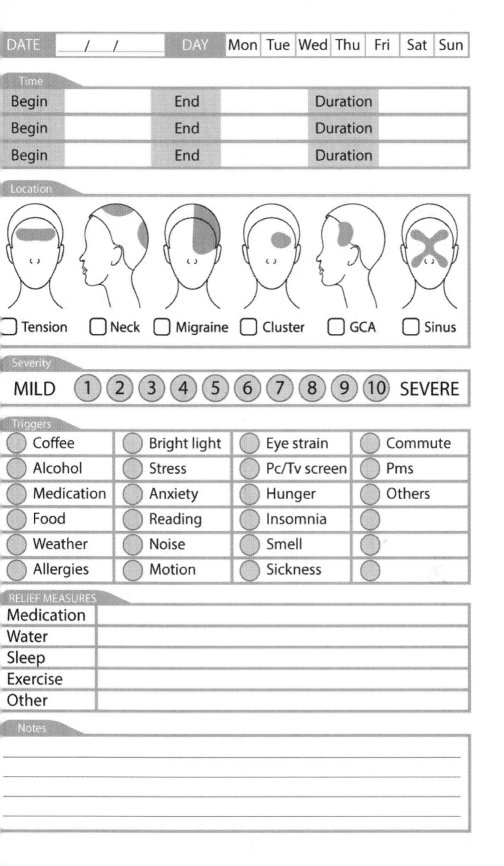

| DATE | / / | DAY | Mon | Tue | Wed | Thu | Fri | Sat | Sun |

Time

Begin		End		Duration	
Begin		End		Duration	
Begin		End		Duration	

Location

☐ Tension   ☐ Neck   ☐ Migraine   ☐ Cluster   ☐ GCA   ☐ Sinus

Severity

MILD ① ② ③ ④ ⑤ ⑥ ⑦ ⑧ ⑨ ⑩ SEVERE

Triggers

○ Coffee	○ Bright light	○ Eye strain	○ Commute
○ Alcohol	○ Stress	○ Pc/Tv screen	○ Pms
○ Medication	○ Anxiety	○ Hunger	○ Others
○ Food	○ Reading	○ Insomnia	○
○ Weather	○ Noise	○ Smell	○
○ Allergies	○ Motion	○ Sickness	○

RELIEF MEASURES

Medication	
Water	
Sleep	
Exercise	
Other	

Notes

_____
_____
_____
_____

DATE	/ /	DAY	Mon	Tue	Wed	Thu	Fri	Sat	Sun

Time

Begin		End		Duration	
Begin		End		Duration	
Begin		End		Duration	

Location

☐ Tension   ☐ Neck   ☐ Migraine   ☐ Cluster   ☐ GCA   ☐ Sinus

Severity

MILD (1) (2) (3) (4) (5) (6) (7) (8) (9) (10) SEVERE

Triggers

○ Coffee	○ Bright light	○ Eye strain	○ Commute
○ Alcohol	○ Stress	○ Pc/Tv screen	○ Pms
○ Medication	○ Anxiety	○ Hunger	○ Others
○ Food	○ Reading	○ Insomnia	○
○ Weather	○ Noise	○ Smell	○
○ Allergies	○ Motion	○ Sickness	○

RELIEF MEASURES

Medication	
Water	
Sleep	
Exercise	
Other	

Notes

DATE	/ /	DAY	Mon	Tue	Wed	Thu	Fri	Sat	Sun

Time

Begin		End		Duration	
Begin		End		Duration	
Begin		End		Duration	

Location

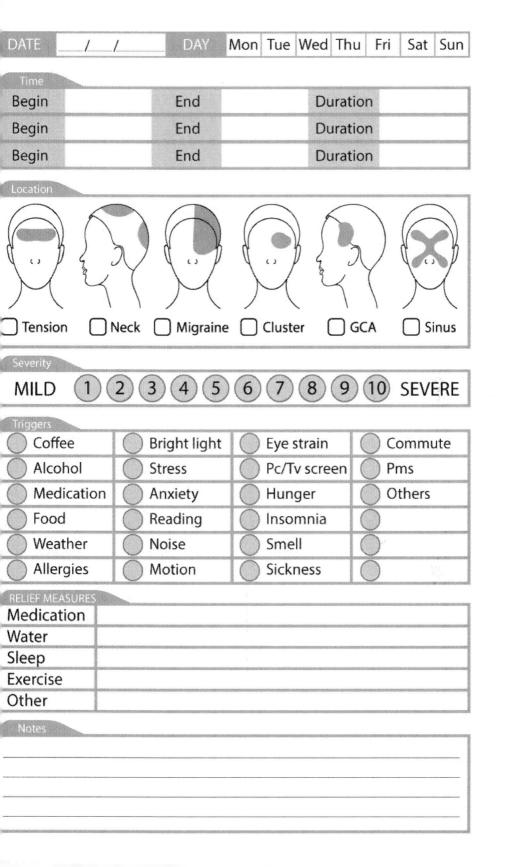

☐ Tension ☐ Neck ☐ Migraine ☐ Cluster ☐ GCA ☐ Sinus

Severity

MILD ① ② ③ ④ ⑤ ⑥ ⑦ ⑧ ⑨ ⑩ SEVERE

Triggers

◯ Coffee	◯ Bright light	◯ Eye strain	◯ Commute
◯ Alcohol	◯ Stress	◯ Pc/Tv screen	◯ Pms
◯ Medication	◯ Anxiety	◯ Hunger	◯ Others
◯ Food	◯ Reading	◯ Insomnia	◯
◯ Weather	◯ Noise	◯ Smell	◯
◯ Allergies	◯ Motion	◯ Sickness	◯

RELIEF MEASURES

Medication	
Water	
Sleep	
Exercise	
Other	

Notes

DATE	/ /	DAY	Mon	Tue	Wed	Thu	Fri	Sat	Sun

Time

Begin		End		Duration	
Begin		End		Duration	
Begin		End		Duration	

Location

☐ Tension   ☐ Neck   ☐ Migraine   ☐ Cluster   ☐ GCA   ☐ Sinus

Severity

MILD ① ② ③ ④ ⑤ ⑥ ⑦ ⑧ ⑨ ⑩ SEVERE

Triggers

○ Coffee	○ Bright light	○ Eye strain	○ Commute
○ Alcohol	○ Stress	○ Pc/Tv screen	○ Pms
○ Medication	○ Anxiety	○ Hunger	○ Others
○ Food	○ Reading	○ Insomnia	○
○ Weather	○ Noise	○ Smell	○
○ Allergies	○ Motion	○ Sickness	○

RELIEF MEASURES

Medication	
Water	
Sleep	
Exercise	
Other	

Notes

DATE	/ /	DAY	Mon	Tue	Wed	Thu	Fri	Sat	Sun

Time

Begin		End		Duration	
Begin		End		Duration	
Begin		End		Duration	

Location

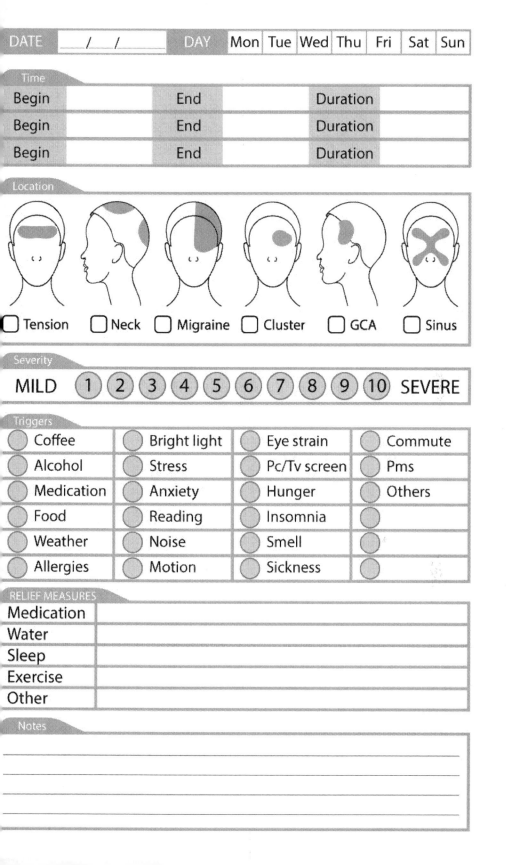

☐ Tension   ☐ Neck   ☐ Migraine   ☐ Cluster   ☐ GCA   ☐ Sinus

Severity

MILD ① ② ③ ④ ⑤ ⑥ ⑦ ⑧ ⑨ ⑩ SEVERE

Triggers

○ Coffee	○ Bright light	○ Eye strain	○ Commute
○ Alcohol	○ Stress	○ Pc/Tv screen	○ Pms
○ Medication	○ Anxiety	○ Hunger	○ Others
○ Food	○ Reading	○ Insomnia	○
○ Weather	○ Noise	○ Smell	○
○ Allergies	○ Motion	○ Sickness	○

RELIEF MEASURES

Medication	
Water	
Sleep	
Exercise	
Other	

Notes

DATE	/ /	DAY	Mon	Tue	Wed	Thu	Fri	Sat	Sun

Time

Begin		End		Duration	
Begin		End		Duration	
Begin		End		Duration	

Location

☐ Tension   ☐ Neck   ☐ Migraine   ☐ Cluster   ☐ GCA   ☐ Sinus

Severity

MILD ① ② ③ ④ ⑤ ⑥ ⑦ ⑧ ⑨ ⑩ SEVERE

Triggers

○ Coffee	○ Bright light	○ Eye strain	○ Commute
○ Alcohol	○ Stress	○ Pc/Tv screen	○ Pms
○ Medication	○ Anxiety	○ Hunger	○ Others
○ Food	○ Reading	○ Insomnia	○
○ Weather	○ Noise	○ Smell	○
○ Allergies	○ Motion	○ Sickness	○

RELIEF MEASURES

Medication	
Water	
Sleep	
Exercise	
Other	

Notes

DATE	/ /	DAY	Mon	Tue	Wed	Thu	Fri	Sat	Sun

Time

Begin		End		Duration	
Begin		End		Duration	
Begin		End		Duration	

Location

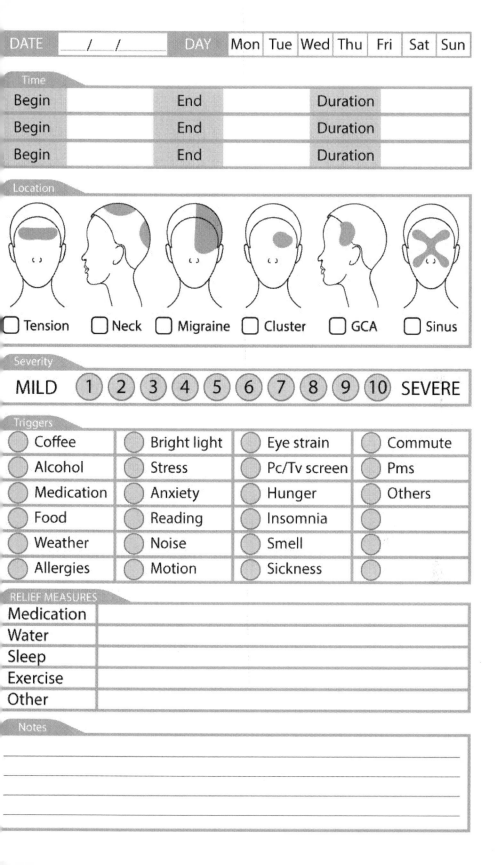

☐ Tension   ☐ Neck   ☐ Migraine   ☐ Cluster   ☐ GCA   ☐ Sinus

Severity

MILD (1) (2) (3) (4) (5) (6) (7) (8) (9) (10) SEVERE

Triggers

○ Coffee	○ Bright light	○ Eye strain	○ Commute
○ Alcohol	○ Stress	○ Pc/Tv screen	○ Pms
○ Medication	○ Anxiety	○ Hunger	○ Others
○ Food	○ Reading	○ Insomnia	○
○ Weather	○ Noise	○ Smell	○
○ Allergies	○ Motion	○ Sickness	○

RELIEF MEASURES

Medication	
Water	
Sleep	
Exercise	
Other	

Notes

DATE	/ /	DAY	Mon	Tue	Wed	Thu	Fri	Sat	Sun

Time

Begin		End		Duration	
Begin		End		Duration	
Begin		End		Duration	

Location

☐ Tension   ☐ Neck   ☐ Migraine   ☐ Cluster   ☐ GCA   ☐ Sinus

Severity

MILD ① ② ③ ④ ⑤ ⑥ ⑦ ⑧ ⑨ ⑩ SEVERE

Triggers

◯ Coffee	◯ Bright light	◯ Eye strain	◯ Commute
◯ Alcohol	◯ Stress	◯ Pc/Tv screen	◯ Pms
◯ Medication	◯ Anxiety	◯ Hunger	◯ Others
◯ Food	◯ Reading	◯ Insomnia	◯
◯ Weather	◯ Noise	◯ Smell	◯
◯ Allergies	◯ Motion	◯ Sickness	◯

RELIEF MEASURES

Medication	
Water	
Sleep	
Exercise	
Other	

Notes

DATE	/ /	DAY	Mon	Tue	Wed	Thu	Fri	Sat	Sun

Time

Begin		End		Duration	
Begin		End		Duration	
Begin		End		Duration	

Location

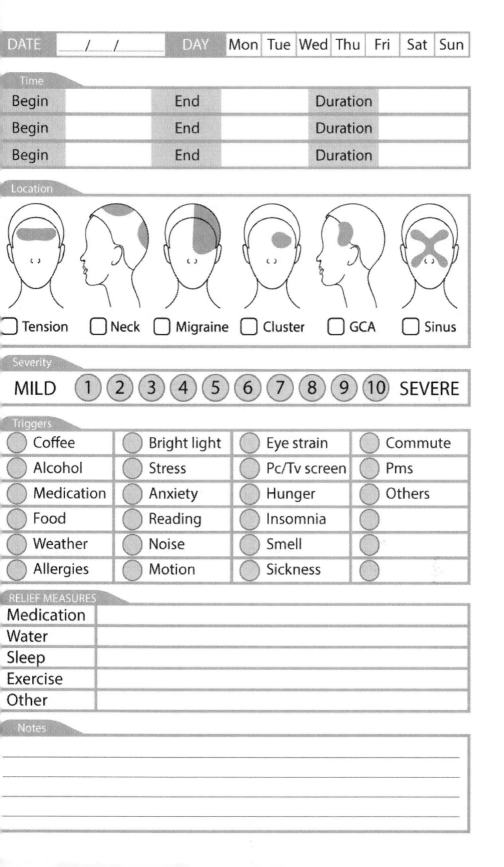

☐ Tension   ☐ Neck   ☐ Migraine   ☐ Cluster   ☐ GCA   ☐ Sinus

Severity

MILD (1) (2) (3) (4) (5) (6) (7) (8) (9) (10) SEVERE

Triggers

◯ Coffee	◯ Bright light	◯ Eye strain	◯ Commute
◯ Alcohol	◯ Stress	◯ Pc/Tv screen	◯ Pms
◯ Medication	◯ Anxiety	◯ Hunger	◯ Others
◯ Food	◯ Reading	◯ Insomnia	◯
◯ Weather	◯ Noise	◯ Smell	◯
◯ Allergies	◯ Motion	◯ Sickness	◯

RELIEF MEASURES

Medication	
Water	
Sleep	
Exercise	
Other	

Notes

| DATE __/__/__ | DAY | Mon | Tue | Wed | Thu | Fri | Sat | Sun |

Time

Begin		End		Duration	
Begin		End		Duration	
Begin		End		Duration	

Location

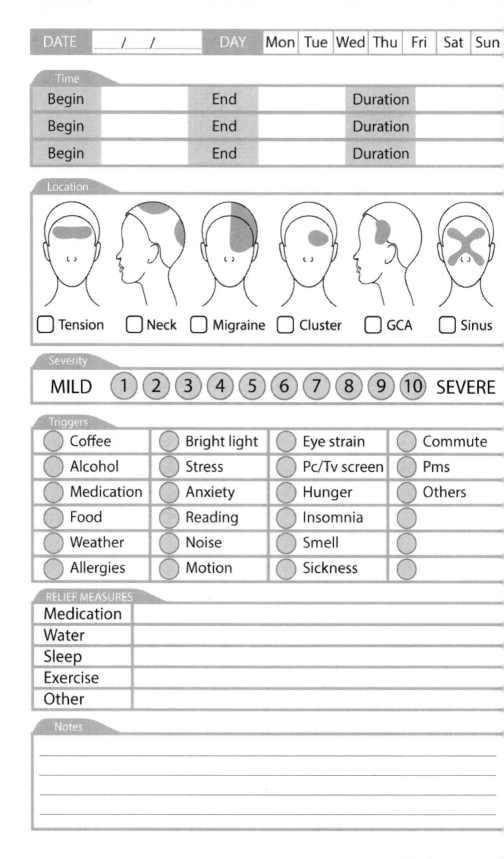

☐ Tension ☐ Neck ☐ Migraine ☐ Cluster ☐ GCA ☐ Sinus

Severity

MILD ① ② ③ ④ ⑤ ⑥ ⑦ ⑧ ⑨ ⑩ SEVERE

Triggers

○ Coffee	○ Bright light	○ Eye strain	○ Commute
○ Alcohol	○ Stress	○ Pc/Tv screen	○ Pms
○ Medication	○ Anxiety	○ Hunger	○ Others
○ Food	○ Reading	○ Insomnia	○
○ Weather	○ Noise	○ Smell	○
○ Allergies	○ Motion	○ Sickness	○

RELIEF MEASURES

Medication	
Water	
Sleep	
Exercise	
Other	

Notes

_____
_____
_____
_____

DATE	/ /	DAY	Mon	Tue	Wed	Thu	Fri	Sat	Sun

Time

Begin		End		Duration	
Begin		End		Duration	
Begin		End		Duration	

Location

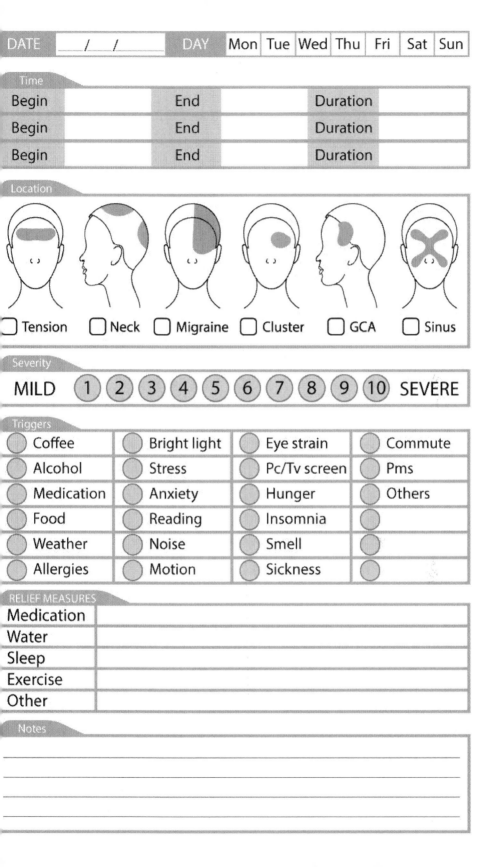

☐ Tension ☐ Neck ☐ Migraine ☐ Cluster ☐ GCA ☐ Sinus

Severity

MILD ① ② ③ ④ ⑤ ⑥ ⑦ ⑧ ⑨ ⑩ SEVERE

Triggers

○ Coffee	○ Bright light	○ Eye strain	○ Commute
○ Alcohol	○ Stress	○ Pc/Tv screen	○ Pms
○ Medication	○ Anxiety	○ Hunger	○ Others
○ Food	○ Reading	○ Insomnia	○
○ Weather	○ Noise	○ Smell	○
○ Allergies	○ Motion	○ Sickness	○

RELIEF MEASURES

Medication	
Water	
Sleep	
Exercise	
Other	

Notes

DATE	/ /	DAY	Mon	Tue	Wed	Thu	Fri	Sat	Sun

Time

Begin		End		Duration	
Begin		End		Duration	
Begin		End		Duration	

Location

☐ Tension   ☐ Neck   ☐ Migraine   ☐ Cluster   ☐ GCA   ☐ Sinus

Severity

MILD ① ② ③ ④ ⑤ ⑥ ⑦ ⑧ ⑨ ⑩ SEVERE

Triggers

○ Coffee	○ Bright light	○ Eye strain	○ Commute
○ Alcohol	○ Stress	○ Pc/Tv screen	○ Pms
○ Medication	○ Anxiety	○ Hunger	○ Others
○ Food	○ Reading	○ Insomnia	○
○ Weather	○ Noise	○ Smell	○
○ Allergies	○ Motion	○ Sickness	○

RELIEF MEASURES

Medication	
Water	
Sleep	
Exercise	
Other	

Notes

DATE	/ /	DAY	Mon	Tue	Wed	Thu	Fri	Sat	Sun

Time

Begin		End		Duration	
Begin		End		Duration	
Begin		End		Duration	

Location

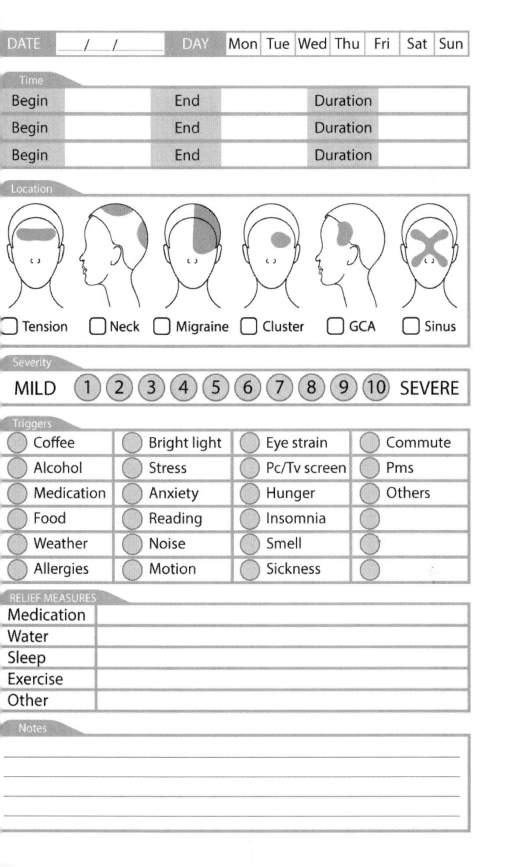

☐ Tension ☐ Neck ☐ Migraine ☐ Cluster ☐ GCA ☐ Sinus

Severity

MILD ① ② ③ ④ ⑤ ⑥ ⑦ ⑧ ⑨ ⑩ SEVERE

Triggers

◯ Coffee	◯ Bright light	◯ Eye strain	◯ Commute
◯ Alcohol	◯ Stress	◯ Pc/Tv screen	◯ Pms
◯ Medication	◯ Anxiety	◯ Hunger	◯ Others
◯ Food	◯ Reading	◯ Insomnia	◯
◯ Weather	◯ Noise	◯ Smell	◯
◯ Allergies	◯ Motion	◯ Sickness	◯

RELIEF MEASURES

Medication	
Water	
Sleep	
Exercise	
Other	

Notes

DATE	/ /	DAY	Mon	Tue	Wed	Thu	Fri	Sat	Sun

Time

Begin		End		Duration	
Begin		End		Duration	
Begin		End		Duration	

Location

☐ Tension ☐ Neck ☐ Migraine ☐ Cluster ☐ GCA ☐ Sinus

Severity

MILD ① ② ③ ④ ⑤ ⑥ ⑦ ⑧ ⑨ ⑩ SEVERE

Triggers

○ Coffee	○ Bright light	○ Eye strain	○ Commute
○ Alcohol	○ Stress	○ Pc/Tv screen	○ Pms
○ Medication	○ Anxiety	○ Hunger	○ Others
○ Food	○ Reading	○ Insomnia	○
○ Weather	○ Noise	○ Smell	○
○ Allergies	○ Motion	○ Sickness	○

RELIEF MEASURES

Medication	
Water	
Sleep	
Exercise	
Other	

Notes

| DATE | / / | DAY | Mon | Tue | Wed | Thu | Fri | Sat | Sun |

Time

Begin		End		Duration	
Begin		End		Duration	
Begin		End		Duration	

Location

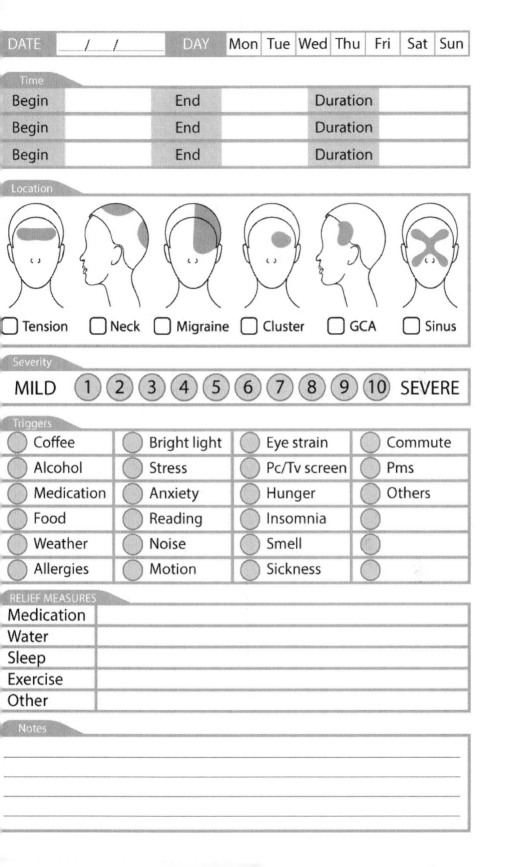

☐ Tension   ☐ Neck   ☐ Migraine   ☐ Cluster   ☐ GCA   ☐ Sinus

Severity

MILD ① ② ③ ④ ⑤ ⑥ ⑦ ⑧ ⑨ ⑩ SEVERE

Triggers

○ Coffee	○ Bright light	○ Eye strain	○ Commute
○ Alcohol	○ Stress	○ Pc/Tv screen	○ Pms
○ Medication	○ Anxiety	○ Hunger	○ Others
○ Food	○ Reading	○ Insomnia	○
○ Weather	○ Noise	○ Smell	○
○ Allergies	○ Motion	○ Sickness	○

RELIEF MEASURES

Medication	
Water	
Sleep	
Exercise	
Other	

Notes

_____
_____
_____
_____

DATE	/ /	DAY	Mon	Tue	Wed	Thu	Fri	Sat	Sun

Time

Begin		End		Duration	
Begin		End		Duration	
Begin		End		Duration	

Location

☐ Tension   ☐ Neck   ☐ Migraine   ☐ Cluster   ☐ GCA   ☐ Sinus

Severity

MILD (1) (2) (3) (4) (5) (6) (7) (8) (9) (10) SEVERE

Triggers

◯ Coffee	◯ Bright light	◯ Eye strain	◯ Commute
◯ Alcohol	◯ Stress	◯ Pc/Tv screen	◯ Pms
◯ Medication	◯ Anxiety	◯ Hunger	◯ Others
◯ Food	◯ Reading	◯ Insomnia	◯
◯ Weather	◯ Noise	◯ Smell	◯
◯ Allergies	◯ Motion	◯ Sickness	◯

RELIEF MEASURES

Medication	
Water	
Sleep	
Exercise	
Other	

Notes

DATE	/ /	DAY	Mon	Tue	Wed	Thu	Fri	Sat	Sun

Time

Begin		End		Duration	
Begin		End		Duration	
Begin		End		Duration	

Location

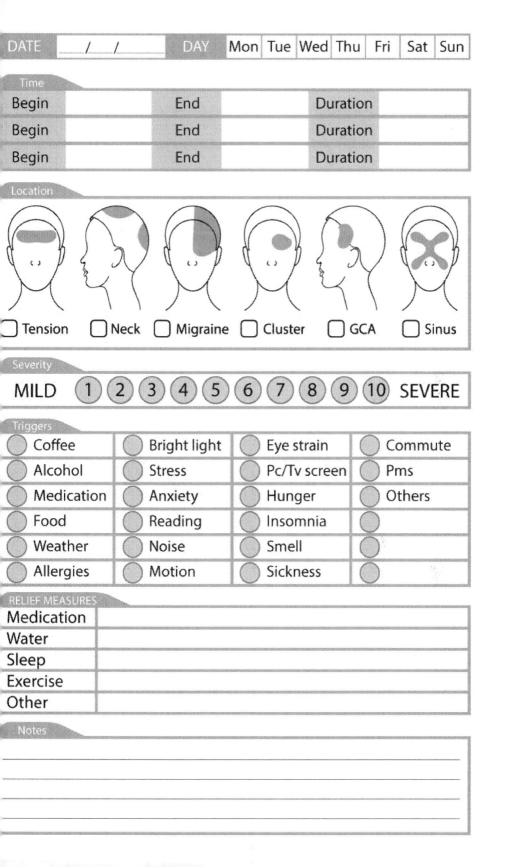

☐ Tension ☐ Neck ☐ Migraine ☐ Cluster ☐ GCA ☐ Sinus

Severity

MILD ① ② ③ ④ ⑤ ⑥ ⑦ ⑧ ⑨ ⑩ SEVERE

Triggers

○ Coffee	○ Bright light	○ Eye strain	○ Commute
○ Alcohol	○ Stress	○ Pc/Tv screen	○ Pms
○ Medication	○ Anxiety	○ Hunger	○ Others
○ Food	○ Reading	○ Insomnia	○
○ Weather	○ Noise	○ Smell	○
○ Allergies	○ Motion	○ Sickness	○

RELIEF MEASURES

Medication	
Water	
Sleep	
Exercise	
Other	

Notes

_____
_____
_____
_____
_____

DATE	/ /	DAY	Mon	Tue	Wed	Thu	Fri	Sat	Sun

Time

Begin		End		Duration	
Begin		End		Duration	
Begin		End		Duration	

Location

☐ Tension   ☐ Neck   ☐ Migraine   ☐ Cluster   ☐ GCA   ☐ Sinus

Severity

MILD ①②③④⑤⑥⑦⑧⑨⑩ SEVERE

Triggers

○ Coffee	○ Bright light	○ Eye strain	○ Commute
○ Alcohol	○ Stress	○ Pc/Tv screen	○ Pms
○ Medication	○ Anxiety	○ Hunger	○ Others
○ Food	○ Reading	○ Insomnia	○
○ Weather	○ Noise	○ Smell	○
○ Allergies	○ Motion	○ Sickness	○

RELIEF MEASURES

Medication	
Water	
Sleep	
Exercise	
Other	

Notes

DATE	/ /	DAY	Mon	Tue	Wed	Thu	Fri	Sat	Sun

Time

Begin		End		Duration	
Begin		End		Duration	
Begin		End		Duration	

Location

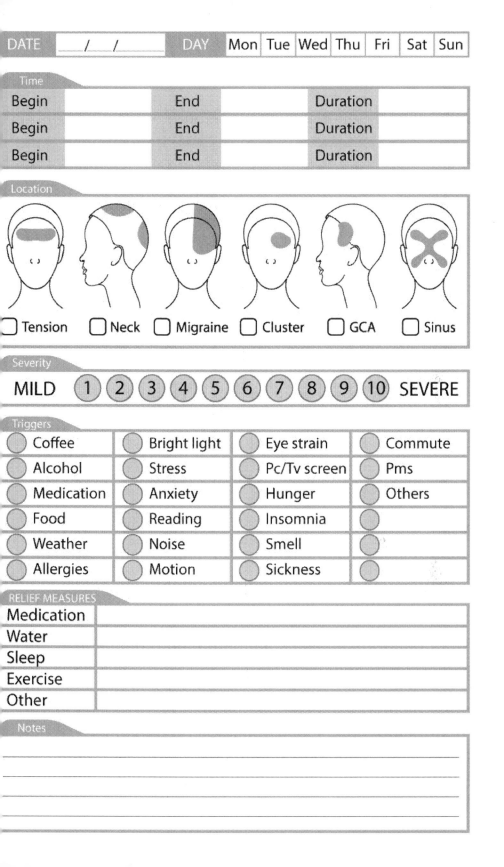

☐ Tension   ☐ Neck   ☐ Migraine   ☐ Cluster   ☐ GCA   ☐ Sinus

Severity

MILD ① ② ③ ④ ⑤ ⑥ ⑦ ⑧ ⑨ ⑩ SEVERE

Triggers

◯ Coffee	◯ Bright light	◯ Eye strain	◯ Commute
◯ Alcohol	◯ Stress	◯ Pc/Tv screen	◯ Pms
◯ Medication	◯ Anxiety	◯ Hunger	◯ Others
◯ Food	◯ Reading	◯ Insomnia	◯
◯ Weather	◯ Noise	◯ Smell	◯
◯ Allergies	◯ Motion	◯ Sickness	◯

RELIEF MEASURES

Medication	
Water	
Sleep	
Exercise	
Other	

Notes

DATE	/ /	DAY	Mon	Tue	Wed	Thu	Fri	Sat	Sun

Time

Begin		End		Duration	
Begin		End		Duration	
Begin		End		Duration	

Location

☐ Tension ☐ Neck ☐ Migraine ☐ Cluster ☐ GCA ☐ Sinus

Severity

MILD ① ② ③ ④ ⑤ ⑥ ⑦ ⑧ ⑨ ⑩ SEVERE

Triggers

○ Coffee	○ Bright light	○ Eye strain	○ Commute
○ Alcohol	○ Stress	○ Pc/Tv screen	○ Pms
○ Medication	○ Anxiety	○ Hunger	○ Others
○ Food	○ Reading	○ Insomnia	○
○ Weather	○ Noise	○ Smell	○
○ Allergies	○ Motion	○ Sickness	○

RELIEF MEASURES

Medication	
Water	
Sleep	
Exercise	
Other	

Notes

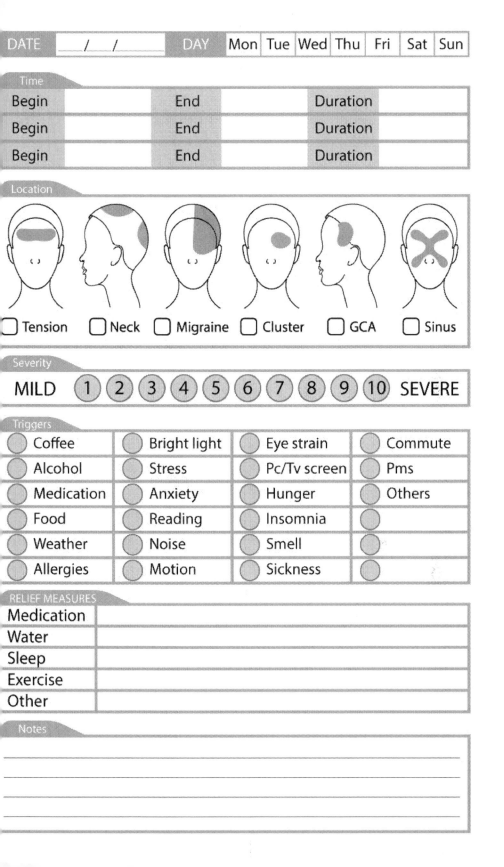

| DATE | / / | DAY | Mon | Tue | Wed | Thu | Fri | Sat | Sun |

Time

Begin		End		Duration	
Begin		End		Duration	
Begin		End		Duration	

Location

☐ Tension ☐ Neck ☐ Migraine ☐ Cluster ☐ GCA ☐ Sinus

Severity

MILD (1) (2) (3) (4) (5) (6) (7) (8) (9) (10) SEVERE

Triggers

○ Coffee	○ Bright light	○ Eye strain	○ Commute
○ Alcohol	○ Stress	○ Pc/Tv screen	○ Pms
○ Medication	○ Anxiety	○ Hunger	○ Others
○ Food	○ Reading	○ Insomnia	○
○ Weather	○ Noise	○ Smell	○
○ Allergies	○ Motion	○ Sickness	○

RELIEF MEASURES

Medication	
Water	
Sleep	
Exercise	
Other	

Notes

DATE	/ /	DAY	Mon	Tue	Wed	Thu	Fri	Sat	Sun

Time

Begin		End		Duration	
Begin		End		Duration	
Begin		End		Duration	

Location

☐ Tension ☐ Neck ☐ Migraine ☐ Cluster ☐ GCA ☐ Sinus

Severity

MILD (1) (2) (3) (4) (5) (6) (7) (8) (9) (10) SEVERE

Triggers

◯ Coffee	◯ Bright light	◯ Eye strain	◯ Commute
◯ Alcohol	◯ Stress	◯ Pc/Tv screen	◯ Pms
◯ Medication	◯ Anxiety	◯ Hunger	◯ Others
◯ Food	◯ Reading	◯ Insomnia	◯
◯ Weather	◯ Noise	◯ Smell	◯
◯ Allergies	◯ Motion	◯ Sickness	◯

RELIEF MEASURES

Medication	
Water	
Sleep	
Exercise	
Other	

Notes

DATE	/ /	DAY	Mon	Tue	Wed	Thu	Fri	Sat	Sun

Time

Begin		End		Duration	
Begin		End		Duration	
Begin		End		Duration	

Location

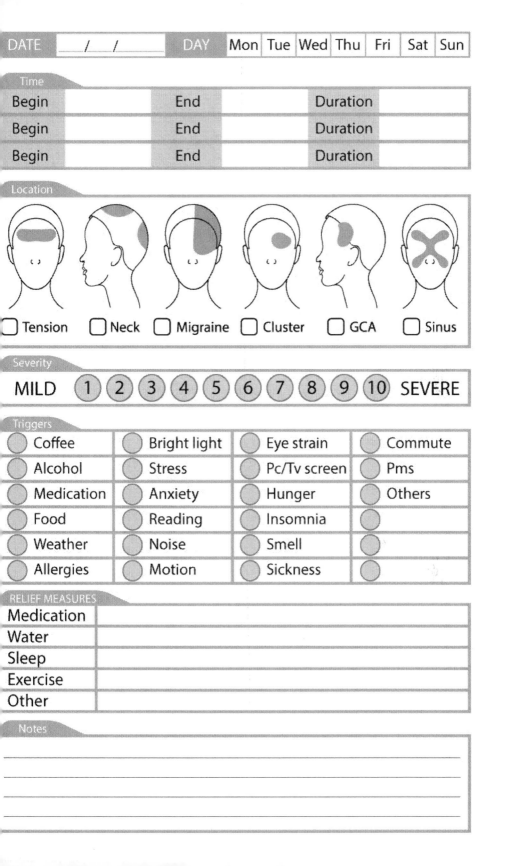

☐ Tension ☐ Neck ☐ Migraine ☐ Cluster ☐ GCA ☐ Sinus

Severity

MILD ① ② ③ ④ ⑤ ⑥ ⑦ ⑧ ⑨ ⑩ SEVERE

Triggers

◯ Coffee	◯ Bright light	◯ Eye strain	◯ Commute
◯ Alcohol	◯ Stress	◯ Pc/Tv screen	◯ Pms
◯ Medication	◯ Anxiety	◯ Hunger	◯ Others
◯ Food	◯ Reading	◯ Insomnia	◯
◯ Weather	◯ Noise	◯ Smell	◯
◯ Allergies	◯ Motion	◯ Sickness	◯

RELIEF MEASURES

Medication	
Water	
Sleep	
Exercise	
Other	

Notes

DATE	/ /	DAY	Mon	Tue	Wed	Thu	Fri	Sat	Sun

Time

Begin		End		Duration	
Begin		End		Duration	
Begin		End		Duration	

Location

☐ Tension ☐ Neck ☐ Migraine ☐ Cluster ☐ GCA ☐ Sinus

Severity

MILD ① ② ③ ④ ⑤ ⑥ ⑦ ⑧ ⑨ ⑩ SEVERE

Triggers

○ Coffee	○ Bright light	○ Eye strain	○ Commute
○ Alcohol	○ Stress	○ Pc/Tv screen	○ Pms
○ Medication	○ Anxiety	○ Hunger	○ Others
○ Food	○ Reading	○ Insomnia	○
○ Weather	○ Noise	○ Smell	○
○ Allergies	○ Motion	○ Sickness	○

RELIEF MEASURES

Medication	
Water	
Sleep	
Exercise	
Other	

Notes

DATE	/ /	DAY	Mon	Tue	Wed	Thu	Fri	Sat	Sun

Time

Begin		End		Duration	
Begin		End		Duration	
Begin		End		Duration	

Location

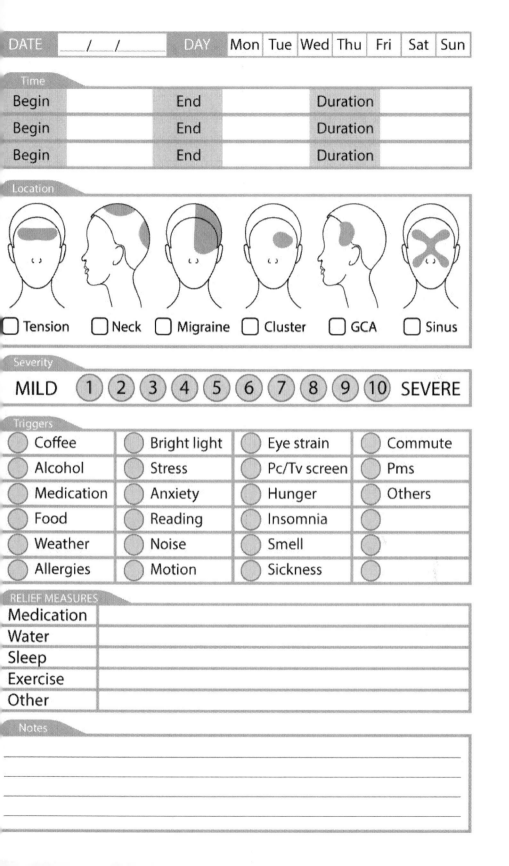

☐ Tension   ☐ Neck   ☐ Migraine   ☐ Cluster   ☐ GCA   ☐ Sinus

Severity

MILD ① ② ③ ④ ⑤ ⑥ ⑦ ⑧ ⑨ ⑩ SEVERE

Triggers

○ Coffee	○ Bright light	○ Eye strain	○ Commute
○ Alcohol	○ Stress	○ Pc/Tv screen	○ Pms
○ Medication	○ Anxiety	○ Hunger	○ Others
○ Food	○ Reading	○ Insomnia	○
○ Weather	○ Noise	○ Smell	○
○ Allergies	○ Motion	○ Sickness	○

RELIEF MEASURES

Medication	
Water	
Sleep	
Exercise	
Other	

Notes

| DATE ___/___/___ | DAY | Mon | Tue | Wed | Thu | Fri | Sat | Sun |

Time

Begin		End		Duration	
Begin		End		Duration	
Begin		End		Duration	

Location

☐ Tension ☐ Neck ☐ Migraine ☐ Cluster ☐ GCA ☐ Sinus

Severity

MILD ① ② ③ ④ ⑤ ⑥ ⑦ ⑧ ⑨ ⑩ SEVERE

Triggers

○ Coffee	○ Bright light	○ Eye strain	○ Commute
○ Alcohol	○ Stress	○ Pc/Tv screen	○ Pms
○ Medication	○ Anxiety	○ Hunger	○ Others
○ Food	○ Reading	○ Insomnia	○
○ Weather	○ Noise	○ Smell	○
○ Allergies	○ Motion	○ Sickness	○

RELIEF MEASURES

Medication	
Water	
Sleep	
Exercise	
Other	

Notes

_____
_____
_____
_____

DATE	/ /	DAY	Mon	Tue	Wed	Thu	Fri	Sat	Sun

Time

Begin		End		Duration	
Begin		End		Duration	
Begin		End		Duration	

Location

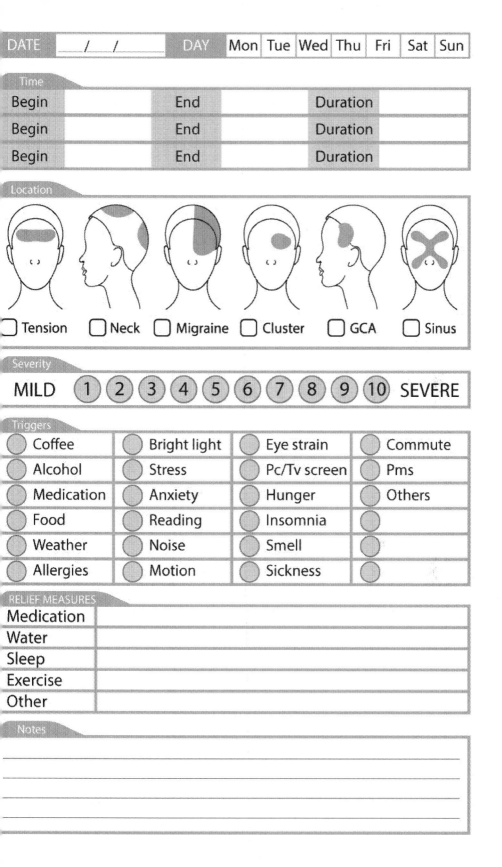

☐ Tension   ☐ Neck   ☐ Migraine   ☐ Cluster   ☐ GCA   ☐ Sinus

Severity

MILD (1) (2) (3) (4) (5) (6) (7) (8) (9) (10) SEVERE

Triggers

○ Coffee	○ Bright light	○ Eye strain	○ Commute
○ Alcohol	○ Stress	○ Pc/Tv screen	○ Pms
○ Medication	○ Anxiety	○ Hunger	○ Others
○ Food	○ Reading	○ Insomnia	○
○ Weather	○ Noise	○ Smell	○
○ Allergies	○ Motion	○ Sickness	○

RELIEF MEASURES

Medication	
Water	
Sleep	
Exercise	
Other	

Notes

_____
_____
_____
_____

DATE	/ /	DAY	Mon	Tue	Wed	Thu	Fri	Sat	Sun

Time

Begin		End		Duration	
Begin		End		Duration	
Begin		End		Duration	

Location

☐ Tension   ☐ Neck   ☐ Migraine   ☐ Cluster   ☐ GCA   ☐ Sinus

Severity

MILD (1) (2) (3) (4) (5) (6) (7) (8) (9) (10) SEVERE

Triggers

◯ Coffee	◯ Bright light	◯ Eye strain	◯ Commute
◯ Alcohol	◯ Stress	◯ Pc/Tv screen	◯ Pms
◯ Medication	◯ Anxiety	◯ Hunger	◯ Others
◯ Food	◯ Reading	◯ Insomnia	◯
◯ Weather	◯ Noise	◯ Smell	◯
◯ Allergies	◯ Motion	◯ Sickness	◯

RELIEF MEASURES

Medication	
Water	
Sleep	
Exercise	
Other	

Notes

DATE	/ /		DAY	Mon	Tue	Wed	Thu	Fri	Sat	Sun

Time

Begin		End		Duration	
Begin		End		Duration	
Begin		End		Duration	

Location

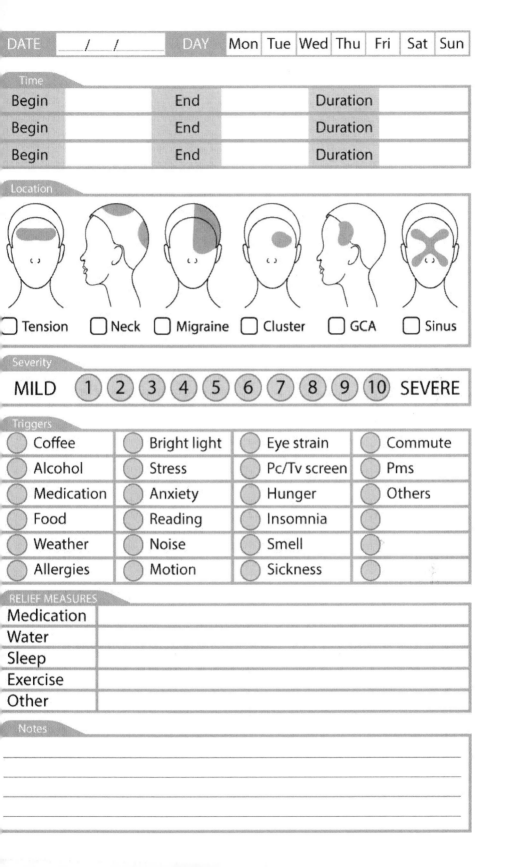

☐ Tension ☐ Neck ☐ Migraine ☐ Cluster ☐ GCA ☐ Sinus

Severity

MILD ①②③④⑤⑥⑦⑧⑨⑩ SEVERE

Triggers

◯ Coffee	◯ Bright light	◯ Eye strain	◯ Commute
◯ Alcohol	◯ Stress	◯ Pc/Tv screen	◯ Pms
◯ Medication	◯ Anxiety	◯ Hunger	◯ Others
◯ Food	◯ Reading	◯ Insomnia	◯
◯ Weather	◯ Noise	◯ Smell	◯
◯ Allergies	◯ Motion	◯ Sickness	◯

RELIEF MEASURES

Medication	
Water	
Sleep	
Exercise	
Other	

Notes

DATE	/ /	DAY	Mon	Tue	Wed	Thu	Fri	Sat	Sun

Time

Begin		End		Duration	
Begin		End		Duration	
Begin		End		Duration	

Location

☐ Tension   ☐ Neck   ☐ Migraine   ☐ Cluster   ☐ GCA   ☐ Sinus

Severity

MILD ① ② ③ ④ ⑤ ⑥ ⑦ ⑧ ⑨ ⑩ SEVERE

Triggers

◯ Coffee	◯ Bright light	◯ Eye strain	◯ Commute
◯ Alcohol	◯ Stress	◯ Pc/Tv screen	◯ Pms
◯ Medication	◯ Anxiety	◯ Hunger	◯ Others
◯ Food	◯ Reading	◯ Insomnia	◯
◯ Weather	◯ Noise	◯ Smell	◯
◯ Allergies	◯ Motion	◯ Sickness	◯

RELIEF MEASURES

Medication	
Water	
Sleep	
Exercise	
Other	

Notes

_____
_____
_____
_____

DATE	/ /	DAY	Mon	Tue	Wed	Thu	Fri	Sat	Sun

Time

Begin		End		Duration	
Begin		End		Duration	
Begin		End		Duration	

Location

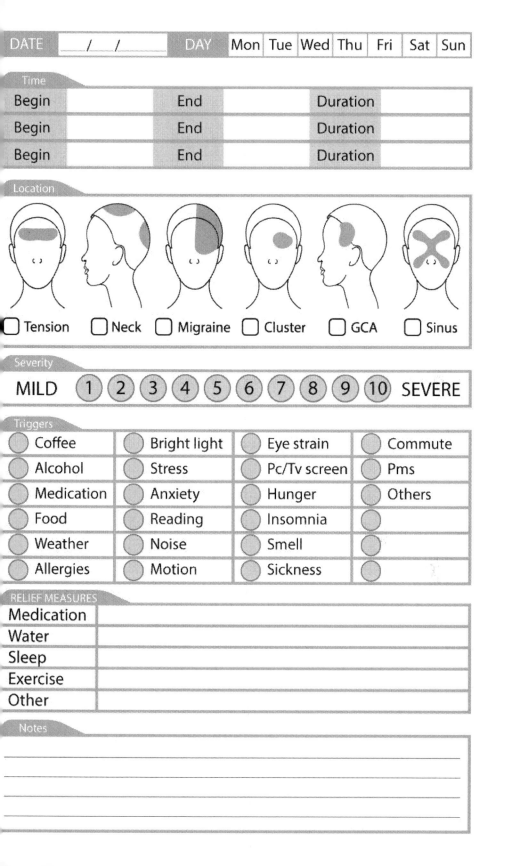

☑ Tension ☐ Neck ☐ Migraine ☐ Cluster ☐ GCA ☐ Sinus

Severity

MILD ① ② ③ ④ ⑤ ⑥ ⑦ ⑧ ⑨ ⑩ SEVERE

Triggers

◯ Coffee	◯ Bright light	◯ Eye strain	◯ Commute
◯ Alcohol	◯ Stress	◯ Pc/Tv screen	◯ Pms
◯ Medication	◯ Anxiety	◯ Hunger	◯ Others
◯ Food	◯ Reading	◯ Insomnia	◯
◯ Weather	◯ Noise	◯ Smell	◯
◯ Allergies	◯ Motion	◯ Sickness	◯

RELIEF MEASURES

Medication	
Water	
Sleep	
Exercise	
Other	

Notes

_____
_____
_____
_____

Time

Begin		End		Duration	
Begin		End		Duration	
Begin		End		Duration	

Location

☐ Tension   ☐ Neck   ☐ Migraine   ☐ Cluster   ☐ GCA   ☐ Sinus

Severity

MILD ① ② ③ ④ ⑤ ⑥ ⑦ ⑧ ⑨ ⑩ SEVERE

Triggers

◯ Coffee	◯ Bright light	◯ Eye strain	◯ Commute
◯ Alcohol	◯ Stress	◯ Pc/Tv screen	◯ Pms
◯ Medication	◯ Anxiety	◯ Hunger	◯ Others
◯ Food	◯ Reading	◯ Insomnia	◯
◯ Weather	◯ Noise	◯ Smell	◯
◯ Allergies	◯ Motion	◯ Sickness	◯

RELIEF MEASURES

Medication	
Water	
Sleep	
Exercise	
Other	

Notes

_____
_____
_____
_____

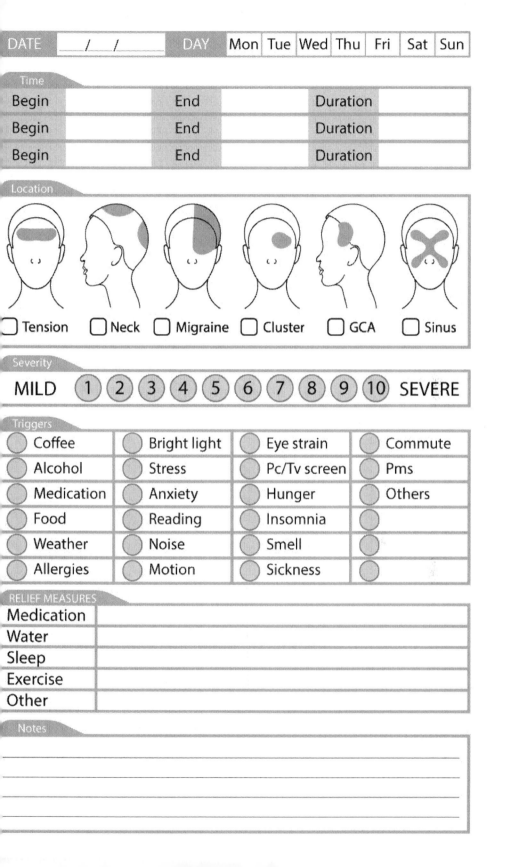

| DATE | / / | DAY | Mon | Tue | Wed | Thu | Fri | Sat | Sun |

Time

Begin		End		Duration	
Begin		End		Duration	
Begin		End		Duration	

Location

☐ Tension   ☐ Neck   ☐ Migraine   ☐ Cluster   ☐ GCA   ☐ Sinus

Severity

MILD ① ② ③ ④ ⑤ ⑥ ⑦ ⑧ ⑨ ⑩ SEVERE

Triggers

◯ Coffee	◯ Bright light	◯ Eye strain	◯ Commute
◯ Alcohol	◯ Stress	◯ Pc/Tv screen	◯ Pms
◯ Medication	◯ Anxiety	◯ Hunger	◯ Others
◯ Food	◯ Reading	◯ Insomnia	◯
◯ Weather	◯ Noise	◯ Smell	◯
◯ Allergies	◯ Motion	◯ Sickness	◯

RELIEF MEASURES

Medication	
Water	
Sleep	
Exercise	
Other	

Notes

DATE	/ /	DAY	Mon	Tue	Wed	Thu	Fri	Sat	Sun

Time

Begin		End		Duration	
Begin		End		Duration	
Begin		End		Duration	

Location

☐ Tension   ☐ Neck   ☐ Migraine   ☐ Cluster   ☐ GCA   ☐ Sinus

Severity

MILD ① ② ③ ④ ⑤ ⑥ ⑦ ⑧ ⑨ ⑩ SEVERE

Triggers

○ Coffee	○ Bright light	○ Eye strain	○ Commute
○ Alcohol	○ Stress	○ Pc/Tv screen	○ Pms
○ Medication	○ Anxiety	○ Hunger	○ Others
○ Food	○ Reading	○ Insomnia	○
○ Weather	○ Noise	○ Smell	○
○ Allergies	○ Motion	○ Sickness	○

RELIEF MEASURES

Medication	
Water	
Sleep	
Exercise	
Other	

Notes

DATE	/ /	DAY	Mon	Tue	Wed	Thu	Fri	Sat	Sun

Time

Begin		End		Duration	
Begin		End		Duration	
Begin		End		Duration	

Location

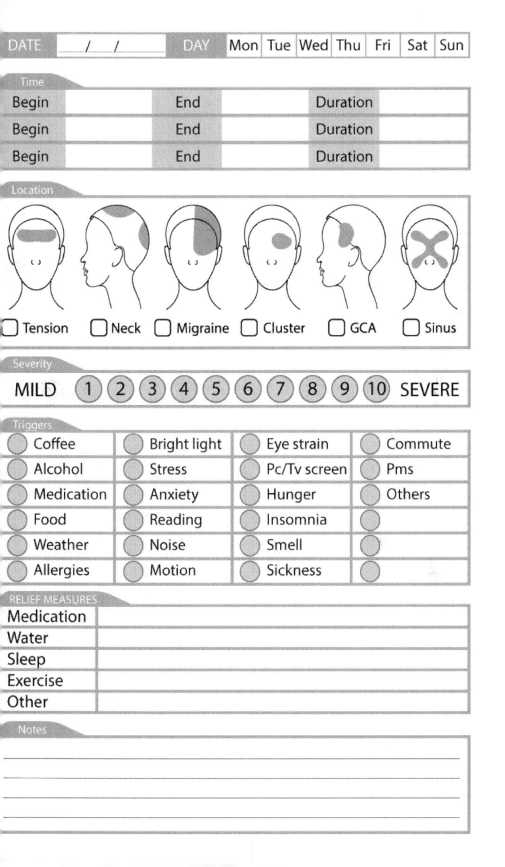

☐ Tension ☐ Neck ☐ Migraine ☐ Cluster ☐ GCA ☐ Sinus

Severity

MILD ① ② ③ ④ ⑤ ⑥ ⑦ ⑧ ⑨ ⑩ SEVERE

Triggers

○ Coffee	○ Bright light	○ Eye strain	○ Commute
○ Alcohol	○ Stress	○ Pc/Tv screen	○ Pms
○ Medication	○ Anxiety	○ Hunger	○ Others
○ Food	○ Reading	○ Insomnia	○
○ Weather	○ Noise	○ Smell	○
○ Allergies	○ Motion	○ Sickness	○

RELIEF MEASURES

Medication	
Water	
Sleep	
Exercise	
Other	

Notes

_____
_____
_____
_____

DATE	/ /		DAY	Mon	Tue	Wed	Thu	Fri	Sat	Sun

Time

Begin		End		Duration	
Begin		End		Duration	
Begin		End		Duration	

Location

☐ Tension   ☐ Neck   ☐ Migraine   ☐ Cluster   ☐ GCA   ☐ Sinus

Severity

MILD ① ② ③ ④ ⑤ ⑥ ⑦ ⑧ ⑨ ⑩ SEVERE

Triggers

Coffee	Bright light	Eye strain	Commute
Alcohol	Stress	Pc/Tv screen	Pms
Medication	Anxiety	Hunger	Others
Food	Reading	Insomnia	
Weather	Noise	Smell	
Allergies	Motion	Sickness	

RELIEF MEASURES

Medication	
Water	
Sleep	
Exercise	
Other	

Notes

DATE	/ /	DAY	Mon	Tue	Wed	Thu	Fri	Sat	Sun

Time

Begin		End		Duration	
Begin		End		Duration	
Begin		End		Duration	

Location

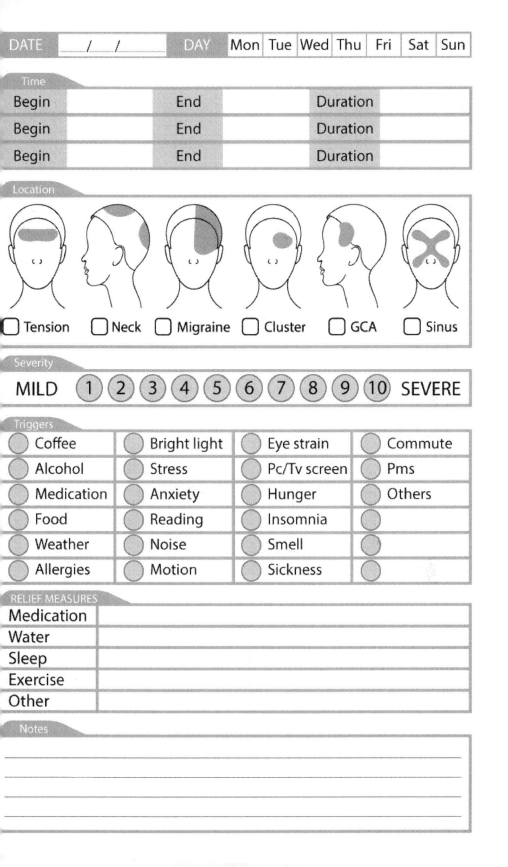

☐ Tension ☐ Neck ☐ Migraine ☐ Cluster ☐ GCA ☐ Sinus

Severity

MILD ① ② ③ ④ ⑤ ⑥ ⑦ ⑧ ⑨ ⑩ SEVERE

Triggers

◯ Coffee	◯ Bright light	◯ Eye strain	◯ Commute
◯ Alcohol	◯ Stress	◯ Pc/Tv screen	◯ Pms
◯ Medication	◯ Anxiety	◯ Hunger	◯ Others
◯ Food	◯ Reading	◯ Insomnia	◯
◯ Weather	◯ Noise	◯ Smell	◯
◯ Allergies	◯ Motion	◯ Sickness	◯

RELIEF MEASURES

Medication	
Water	
Sleep	
Exercise	
Other	

Notes

_____
_____
_____
_____

DATE	/ /	DAY	Mon	Tue	Wed	Thu	Fri	Sat	Sun

Time

Begin		End		Duration	
Begin		End		Duration	
Begin		End		Duration	

Location

☐ Tension   ☐ Neck   ☐ Migraine   ☐ Cluster   ☐ GCA   ☐ Sinus

Severity

MILD (1) (2) (3) (4) (5) (6) (7) (8) (9) (10) SEVERE

Triggers

○ Coffee	○ Bright light	○ Eye strain	○ Commute
○ Alcohol	○ Stress	○ Pc/Tv screen	○ Pms
○ Medication	○ Anxiety	○ Hunger	○ Others
○ Food	○ Reading	○ Insomnia	○
○ Weather	○ Noise	○ Smell	○
○ Allergies	○ Motion	○ Sickness	○

RELIEF MEASURES

Medication	
Water	
Sleep	
Exercise	
Other	

Notes

DATE	/ /	DAY	Mon	Tue	Wed	Thu	Fri	Sat	Sun

Time

Begin		End		Duration	
Begin		End		Duration	
Begin		End		Duration	

Location

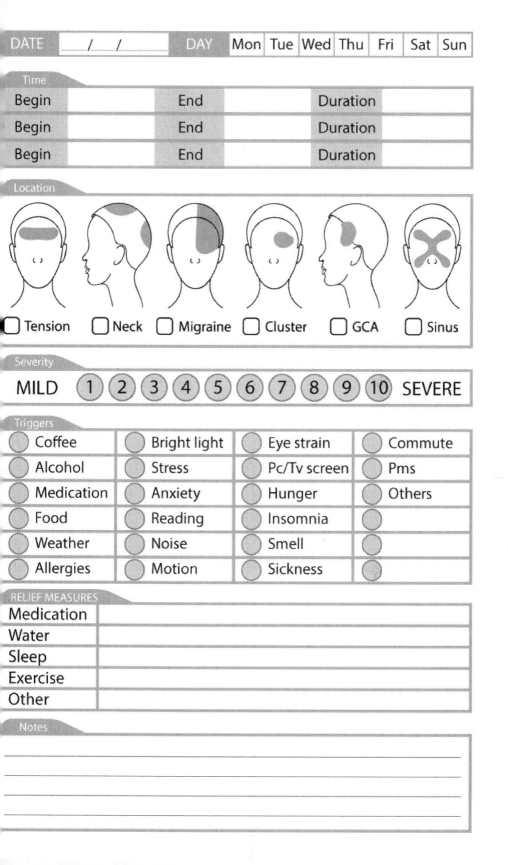

☐ Tension ☐ Neck ☐ Migraine ☐ Cluster ☐ GCA ☐ Sinus

Severity

MILD ①②③④⑤⑥⑦⑧⑨⑩ SEVERE

Triggers

◯ Coffee	◯ Bright light	◯ Eye strain	◯ Commute
◯ Alcohol	◯ Stress	◯ Pc/Tv screen	◯ Pms
◯ Medication	◯ Anxiety	◯ Hunger	◯ Others
◯ Food	◯ Reading	◯ Insomnia	◯
◯ Weather	◯ Noise	◯ Smell	◯
◯ Allergies	◯ Motion	◯ Sickness	◯

RELIEF MEASURES

Medication	
Water	
Sleep	
Exercise	
Other	

Notes

DATE	/ /	DAY	Mon	Tue	Wed	Thu	Fri	Sat	Sun

Time

Begin		End		Duration	
Begin		End		Duration	
Begin		End		Duration	

Location

☐ Tension ☐ Neck ☐ Migraine ☐ Cluster ☐ GCA ☐ Sinus

Severity

MILD ① ② ③ ④ ⑤ ⑥ ⑦ ⑧ ⑨ ⑩ SEVERE

Triggers

○ Coffee	○ Bright light	○ Eye strain	○ Commute
○ Alcohol	○ Stress	○ Pc/Tv screen	○ Pms
○ Medication	○ Anxiety	○ Hunger	○ Others
○ Food	○ Reading	○ Insomnia	○
○ Weather	○ Noise	○ Smell	○
○ Allergies	○ Motion	○ Sickness	○

RELIEF MEASURES

Medication	
Water	
Sleep	
Exercise	
Other	

Notes

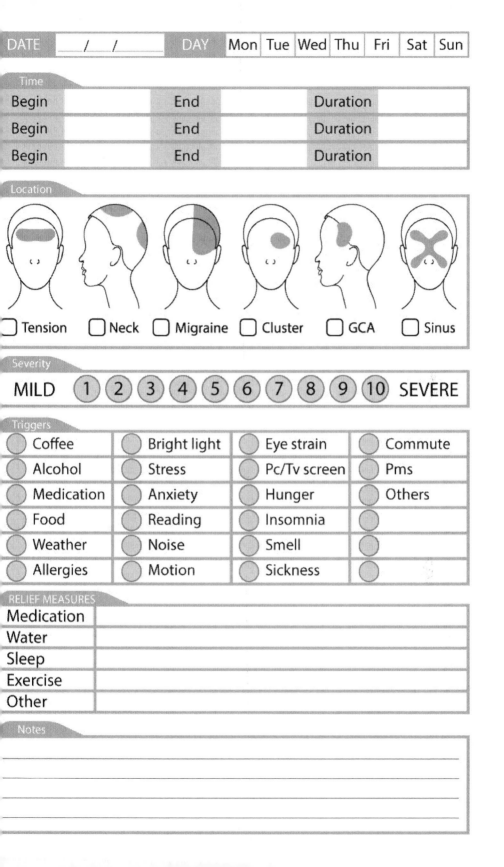

DATE	/ /	DAY	Mon	Tue	Wed	Thu	Fri	Sat	Sun

Time

Begin		End		Duration	
Begin		End		Duration	
Begin		End		Duration	

Location

☐ Tension ☐ Neck ☐ Migraine ☐ Cluster ☐ GCA ☐ Sinus

Severity

MILD ① ② ③ ④ ⑤ ⑥ ⑦ ⑧ ⑨ ⑩ SEVERE

Triggers

○ Coffee	○ Bright light	○ Eye strain	○ Commute
○ Alcohol	○ Stress	○ Pc/Tv screen	○ Pms
○ Medication	○ Anxiety	○ Hunger	○ Others
○ Food	○ Reading	○ Insomnia	○
○ Weather	○ Noise	○ Smell	○
○ Allergies	○ Motion	○ Sickness	○

RELIEF MEASURES

Medication	
Water	
Sleep	
Exercise	
Other	

Notes

DATE	/ /	DAY	Mon	Tue	Wed	Thu	Fri	Sat	Sun

Time

Begin		End		Duration	
Begin		End		Duration	
Begin		End		Duration	

Location

- ☐ Tension
- ☐ Neck
- ☐ Migraine
- ☐ Cluster
- ☐ GCA
- ☐ Sinus

Severity

MILD ① ② ③ ④ ⑤ ⑥ ⑦ ⑧ ⑨ ⑩ SEVERE

Triggers

○ Coffee	○ Bright light	○ Eye strain	○ Commute
○ Alcohol	○ Stress	○ Pc/Tv screen	○ Pms
○ Medication	○ Anxiety	○ Hunger	○ Others
○ Food	○ Reading	○ Insomnia	○
○ Weather	○ Noise	○ Smell	○
○ Allergies	○ Motion	○ Sickness	○

RELIEF MEASURES

Medication	
Water	
Sleep	
Exercise	
Other	

Notes

DATE	/ /	DAY	Mon	Tue	Wed	Thu	Fri	Sat	Sun

Time

Begin		End		Duration	
Begin		End		Duration	
Begin		End		Duration	

Location

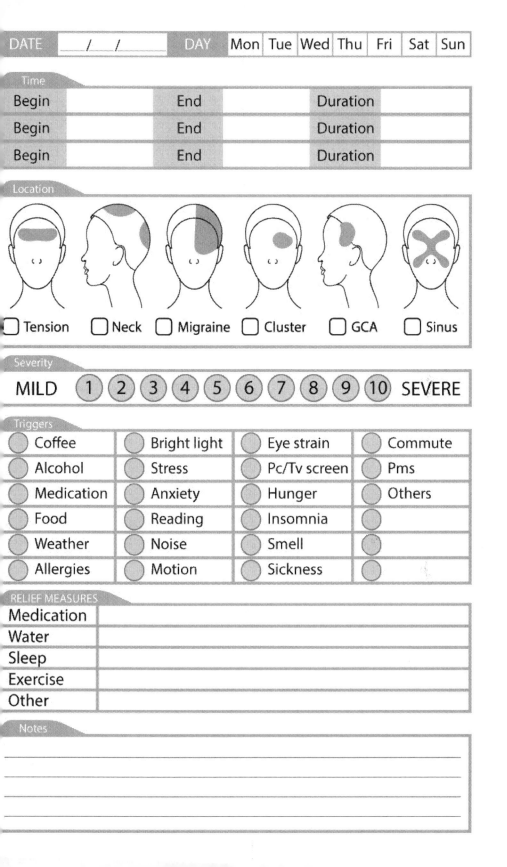

☐ Tension ☐ Neck ☐ Migraine ☐ Cluster ☐ GCA ☐ Sinus

Severity

MILD ① ② ③ ④ ⑤ ⑥ ⑦ ⑧ ⑨ ⑩ SEVERE

Triggers

◯ Coffee	◯ Bright light	◯ Eye strain	◯ Commute
◯ Alcohol	◯ Stress	◯ Pc/Tv screen	◯ Pms
◯ Medication	◯ Anxiety	◯ Hunger	◯ Others
◯ Food	◯ Reading	◯ Insomnia	◯
◯ Weather	◯ Noise	◯ Smell	◯
◯ Allergies	◯ Motion	◯ Sickness	◯

RELIEF MEASURES

Medication	
Water	
Sleep	
Exercise	
Other	

Notes

_____
_____
_____
_____

DATE _____ / _____ / _____		DAY	Mon	Tue	Wed	Thu	Fri	Sat	Sun

Time

Begin		End		Duration	
Begin		End		Duration	
Begin		End		Duration	

Location

☐ Tension ☐ Neck ☐ Migraine ☐ Cluster ☐ GCA ☐ Sinus

Severity

MILD (1) (2) (3) (4) (5) (6) (7) (8) (9) (10) SEVERE

Triggers

◯ Coffee	◯ Bright light	◯ Eye strain	◯ Commute
◯ Alcohol	◯ Stress	◯ Pc/Tv screen	◯ Pms
◯ Medication	◯ Anxiety	◯ Hunger	◯ Others
◯ Food	◯ Reading	◯ Insomnia	◯
◯ Weather	◯ Noise	◯ Smell	◯
◯ Allergies	◯ Motion	◯ Sickness	◯

RELIEF MEASURES

Medication	
Water	
Sleep	
Exercise	
Other	

Notes

DATE	/ /	DAY	Mon	Tue	Wed	Thu	Fri	Sat	Sun

Time

Begin		End		Duration	
Begin		End		Duration	
Begin		End		Duration	

Location

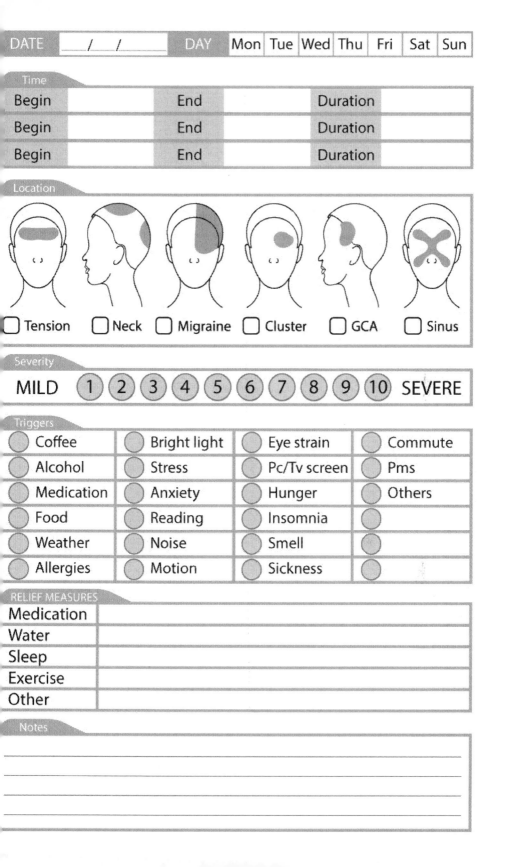

☐ Tension ☐ Neck ☐ Migraine ☐ Cluster ☐ GCA ☐ Sinus

Severity

MILD ① ② ③ ④ ⑤ ⑥ ⑦ ⑧ ⑨ ⑩ SEVERE

Triggers

○ Coffee	○ Bright light	○ Eye strain	○ Commute
○ Alcohol	○ Stress	○ Pc/Tv screen	○ Pms
○ Medication	○ Anxiety	○ Hunger	○ Others
○ Food	○ Reading	○ Insomnia	○
○ Weather	○ Noise	○ Smell	○
○ Allergies	○ Motion	○ Sickness	○

RELIEF MEASURES

Medication	
Water	
Sleep	
Exercise	
Other	

Notes

_____
_____
_____
_____

| DATE | / / | | DAY | Mon | Tue | Wed | Thu | Fri | Sat | Sun |

Begin		End		Duration	
Begin		End		Duration	
Begin		End		Duration	

Location

☐ Tension ☐ Neck ☐ Migraine ☐ Cluster ☐ GCA ☐ Sinus

Severity

MILD ① ② ③ ④ ⑤ ⑥ ⑦ ⑧ ⑨ ⑩ SEVERE

Triggers

○ Coffee	○ Bright light	○ Eye strain	○ Commute
○ Alcohol	○ Stress	○ Pc/Tv screen	○ Pms
○ Medication	○ Anxiety	○ Hunger	○ Others
○ Food	○ Reading	○ Insomnia	○
○ Weather	○ Noise	○ Smell	○
○ Allergies	○ Motion	○ Sickness	○

RELIEF MEASURES

Medication	
Water	
Sleep	
Exercise	
Other	

Notes

_____
_____
_____
_____

DATE	/ /	DAY	Mon	Tue	Wed	Thu	Fri	Sat	Sun

Time

Begin		End		Duration	
Begin		End		Duration	
Begin		End		Duration	

Location

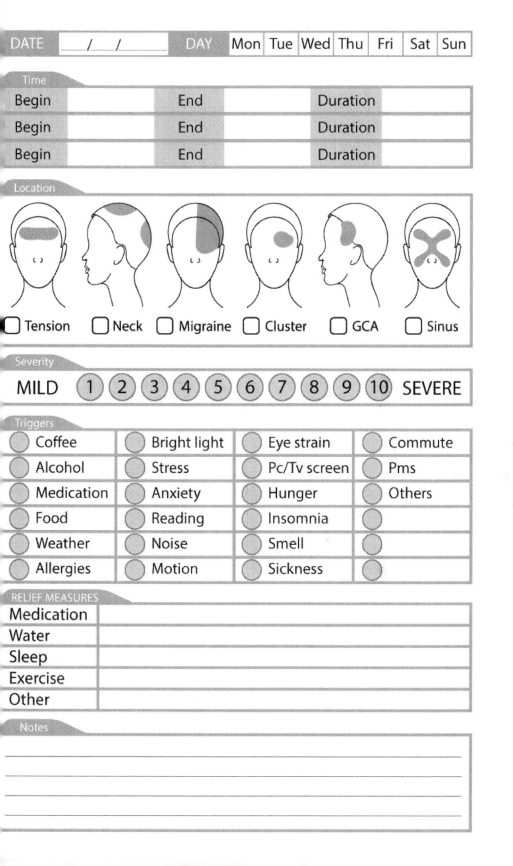

☐ Tension ☐ Neck ☐ Migraine ☐ Cluster ☐ GCA ☐ Sinus

Severity

MILD (1) (2) (3) (4) (5) (6) (7) (8) (9) (10) SEVERE

Triggers

◯ Coffee	◯ Bright light	◯ Eye strain	◯ Commute
◯ Alcohol	◯ Stress	◯ Pc/Tv screen	◯ Pms
◯ Medication	◯ Anxiety	◯ Hunger	◯ Others
◯ Food	◯ Reading	◯ Insomnia	◯
◯ Weather	◯ Noise	◯ Smell	◯
◯ Allergies	◯ Motion	◯ Sickness	◯

RELIEF MEASURES

Medication	
Water	
Sleep	
Exercise	
Other	

Notes

DATE	/ /	DAY	Mon	Tue	Wed	Thu	Fri	Sat	Sun

Time

Begin		End		Duration	
Begin		End		Duration	
Begin		End		Duration	

Location

☐ Tension   ☐ Neck   ☐ Migraine   ☐ Cluster   ☐ GCA   ☐ Sinus

Severity

MILD ① ② ③ ④ ⑤ ⑥ ⑦ ⑧ ⑨ ⑩ SEVERE

Triggers

○ Coffee	○ Bright light	○ Eye strain	○ Commute
○ Alcohol	○ Stress	○ Pc/Tv screen	○ Pms
○ Medication	○ Anxiety	○ Hunger	○ Others
○ Food	○ Reading	○ Insomnia	○
○ Weather	○ Noise	○ Smell	○
○ Allergies	○ Motion	○ Sickness	○

RELIEF MEASURES

Medication	
Water	
Sleep	
Exercise	
Other	

Notes

_____
_____
_____
_____

DATE	/ /	DAY	Mon	Tue	Wed	Thu	Fri	Sat	Sun

Time

Begin		End		Duration	
Begin		End		Duration	
Begin		End		Duration	

Location

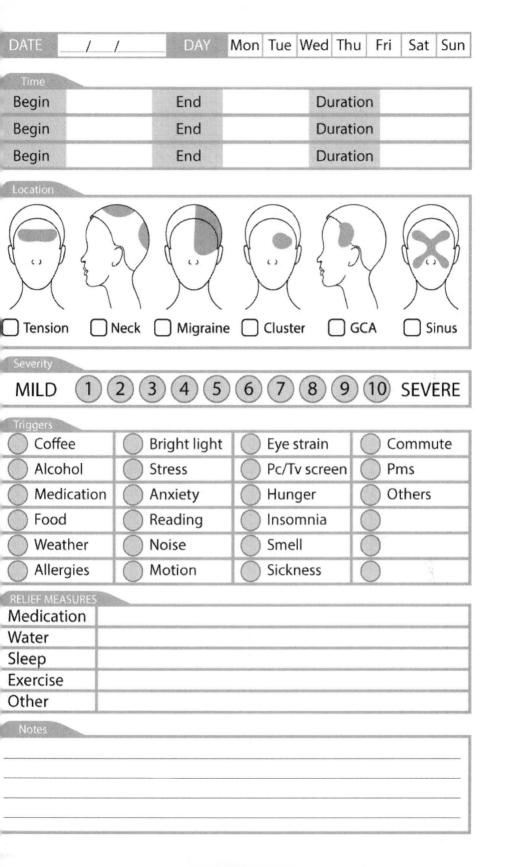

☐ Tension ☐ Neck ☐ Migraine ☐ Cluster ☐ GCA ☐ Sinus

Severity

MILD (1) (2) (3) (4) (5) (6) (7) (8) (9) (10) SEVERE

Triggers

◯ Coffee	◯ Bright light	◯ Eye strain	◯ Commute
◯ Alcohol	◯ Stress	◯ Pc/Tv screen	◯ Pms
◯ Medication	◯ Anxiety	◯ Hunger	◯ Others
◯ Food	◯ Reading	◯ Insomnia	◯
◯ Weather	◯ Noise	◯ Smell	◯
◯ Allergies	◯ Motion	◯ Sickness	◯

RELIEF MEASURES

Medication	
Water	
Sleep	
Exercise	
Other	

Notes

_____
_____
_____
_____
_____

DATE	/ /	DAY	Mon	Tue	Wed	Thu	Fri	Sat	Sun

Time

Begin		End		Duration	
Begin		End		Duration	
Begin		End		Duration	

Location

☐ Tension   ☐ Neck   ☐ Migraine   ☐ Cluster   ☐ GCA   ☐ Sinus

Severity

MILD ① ② ③ ④ ⑤ ⑥ ⑦ ⑧ ⑨ ⑩ SEVERE

Triggers

◯ Coffee	◯ Bright light	◯ Eye strain	◯ Commute
◯ Alcohol	◯ Stress	◯ Pc/Tv screen	◯ Pms
◯ Medication	◯ Anxiety	◯ Hunger	◯ Others
◯ Food	◯ Reading	◯ Insomnia	◯
◯ Weather	◯ Noise	◯ Smell	◯
◯ Allergies	◯ Motion	◯ Sickness	◯

RELIEF MEASURES

Medication	
Water	
Sleep	
Exercise	
Other	

Notes

DATE	/ /	DAY	Mon	Tue	Wed	Thu	Fri	Sat	Sun

Time

Begin		End		Duration	
Begin		End		Duration	
Begin		End		Duration	

Location

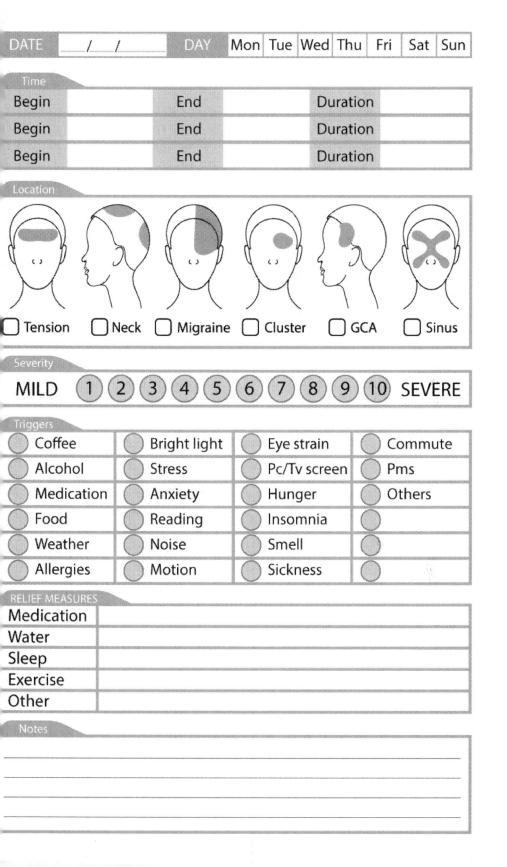

☐ Tension ☐ Neck ☐ Migraine ☐ Cluster ☐ GCA ☐ Sinus

Severity

MILD ① ② ③ ④ ⑤ ⑥ ⑦ ⑧ ⑨ ⑩ SEVERE

Triggers

○ Coffee	○ Bright light	○ Eye strain	○ Commute
○ Alcohol	○ Stress	○ Pc/Tv screen	○ Pms
○ Medication	○ Anxiety	○ Hunger	○ Others
○ Food	○ Reading	○ Insomnia	○
○ Weather	○ Noise	○ Smell	○
○ Allergies	○ Motion	○ Sickness	○

RELIEF MEASURES

Medication	
Water	
Sleep	
Exercise	
Other	

Notes

_____
_____
_____
_____

DATE	/ /	DAY	Mon	Tue	Wed	Thu	Fri	Sat	Sun

Time

Begin		End		Duration	
Begin		End		Duration	
Begin		End		Duration	

Location

☐ Tension	☐ Neck	☐ Migraine	☐ Cluster	☐ GCA	☐ Sinus

Severity

MILD ① ② ③ ④ ⑤ ⑥ ⑦ ⑧ ⑨ ⑩ SEVERE

Triggers

◯ Coffee	◯ Bright light	◯ Eye strain	◯ Commute
◯ Alcohol	◯ Stress	◯ Pc/Tv screen	◯ Pms
◯ Medication	◯ Anxiety	◯ Hunger	◯ Others
◯ Food	◯ Reading	◯ Insomnia	◯
◯ Weather	◯ Noise	◯ Smell	◯
◯ Allergies	◯ Motion	◯ Sickness	◯

RELIEF MEASURES

Medication	
Water	
Sleep	
Exercise	
Other	

Notes

DATE	/ /	DAY	Mon	Tue	Wed	Thu	Fri	Sat	Sun

Time

Begin		End		Duration	
Begin		End		Duration	
Begin		End		Duration	

Location

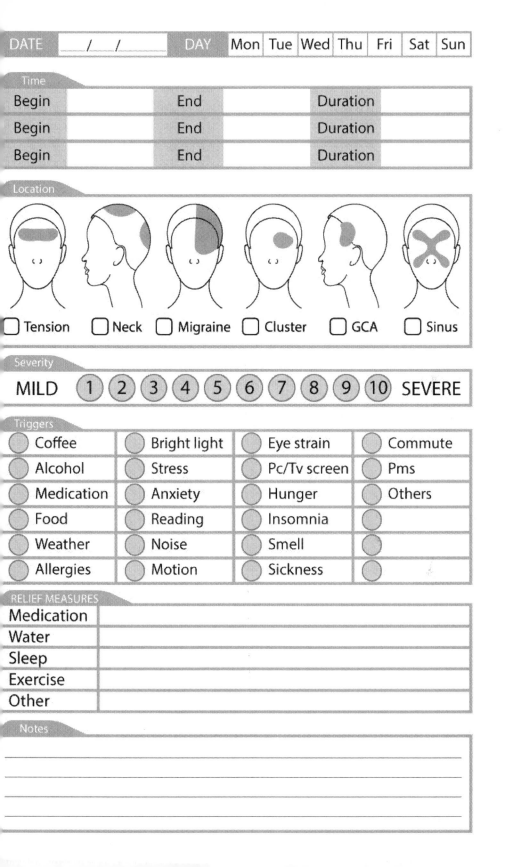

☐ Tension ☐ Neck ☐ Migraine ☐ Cluster ☐ GCA ☐ Sinus

Severity

MILD ① ② ③ ④ ⑤ ⑥ ⑦ ⑧ ⑨ ⑩ SEVERE

Triggers

◯ Coffee	◯ Bright light	◯ Eye strain	◯ Commute
◯ Alcohol	◯ Stress	◯ Pc/Tv screen	◯ Pms
◯ Medication	◯ Anxiety	◯ Hunger	◯ Others
◯ Food	◯ Reading	◯ Insomnia	◯
◯ Weather	◯ Noise	◯ Smell	◯
◯ Allergies	◯ Motion	◯ Sickness	◯

RELIEF MEASURES

Medication	
Water	
Sleep	
Exercise	
Other	

Notes

DATE	/ /	DAY	Mon	Tue	Wed	Thu	Fri	Sat	Sun

Time

Begin		End		Duration	
Begin		End		Duration	
Begin		End		Duration	

Location

☐ Tension   ☐ Neck   ☐ Migraine   ☐ Cluster   ☐ GCA   ☐ Sinus

Severity

MILD ① ② ③ ④ ⑤ ⑥ ⑦ ⑧ ⑨ ⑩ SEVERE

Triggers

◯ Coffee	◯ Bright light	◯ Eye strain	◯ Commute
◯ Alcohol	◯ Stress	◯ Pc/Tv screen	◯ Pms
◯ Medication	◯ Anxiety	◯ Hunger	◯ Others
◯ Food	◯ Reading	◯ Insomnia	◯
◯ Weather	◯ Noise	◯ Smell	◯
◯ Allergies	◯ Motion	◯ Sickness	◯

RELIEF MEASURES

Medication	
Water	
Sleep	
Exercise	
Other	

Notes

DATE	/ /	DAY	Mon	Tue	Wed	Thu	Fri	Sat	Sun

Time

Begin		End		Duration	
Begin		End		Duration	
Begin		End		Duration	

Location

☐ Tension   ☐ Neck   ☐ Migraine   ☐ Cluster   ☐ GCA   ☐ Sinus

Severity

MILD ① ② ③ ④ ⑤ ⑥ ⑦ ⑧ ⑨ ⑩ SEVERE

Triggers

○ Coffee	○ Bright light	○ Eye strain	○ Commute
○ Alcohol	○ Stress	○ Pc/Tv screen	○ Pms
○ Medication	○ Anxiety	○ Hunger	○ Others
○ Food	○ Reading	○ Insomnia	○
○ Weather	○ Noise	○ Smell	○
○ Allergies	○ Motion	○ Sickness	○

RELIEF MEASURES

Medication	
Water	
Sleep	
Exercise	
Other	

Notes

_____
_____
_____
_____

| DATE | / / | DAY | Mon | Tue | Wed | Thu | Fri | Sat | Sun |

Time

Begin		End		Duration	
Begin		End		Duration	
Begin		End		Duration	

Location

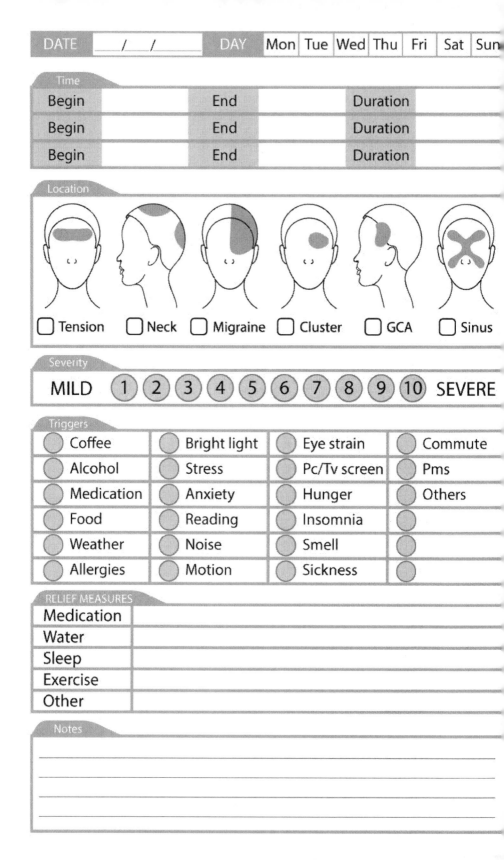

☐ Tension ☐ Neck ☐ Migraine ☐ Cluster ☐ GCA ☐ Sinus

Severity

MILD ① ② ③ ④ ⑤ ⑥ ⑦ ⑧ ⑨ ⑩ SEVERE

Triggers

○ Coffee	○ Bright light	○ Eye strain	○ Commute
○ Alcohol	○ Stress	○ Pc/Tv screen	○ Pms
○ Medication	○ Anxiety	○ Hunger	○ Others
○ Food	○ Reading	○ Insomnia	○
○ Weather	○ Noise	○ Smell	○
○ Allergies	○ Motion	○ Sickness	○

RELIEF MEASURES

Medication	
Water	
Sleep	
Exercise	
Other	

Notes

_____
_____
_____
_____

DATE	/ /	DAY	Mon	Tue	Wed	Thu	Fri	Sat	Sun

Time

Begin		End		Duration	
Begin		End		Duration	
Begin		End		Duration	

Location

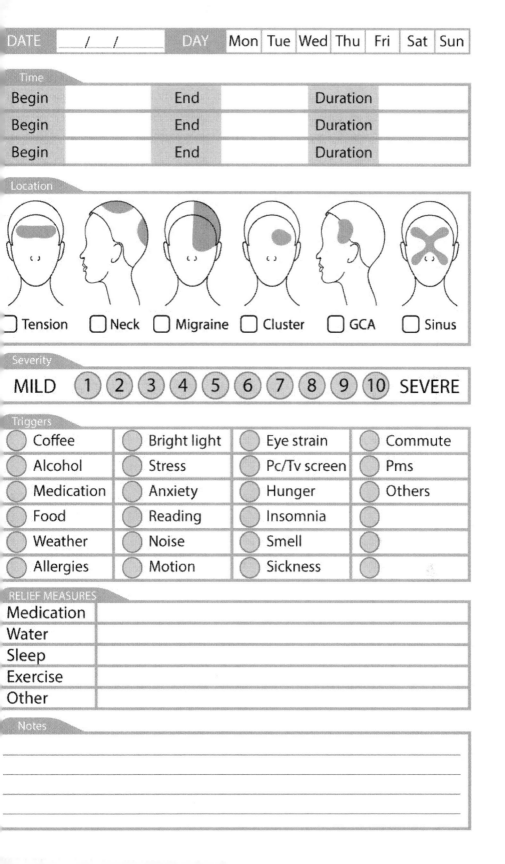

☐ Tension   ☐ Neck   ☐ Migraine   ☐ Cluster   ☐ GCA   ☐ Sinus

Severity

MILD ① ② ③ ④ ⑤ ⑥ ⑦ ⑧ ⑨ ⑩ SEVERE

Triggers

◯ Coffee	◯ Bright light	◯ Eye strain	◯ Commute
◯ Alcohol	◯ Stress	◯ Pc/Tv screen	◯ Pms
◯ Medication	◯ Anxiety	◯ Hunger	◯ Others
◯ Food	◯ Reading	◯ Insomnia	◯
◯ Weather	◯ Noise	◯ Smell	◯
◯ Allergies	◯ Motion	◯ Sickness	◯

RELIEF MEASURES

Medication	
Water	
Sleep	
Exercise	
Other	

Notes

| DATE | / / | DAY | Mon | Tue | Wed | Thu | Fri | Sat | Sun |

Time

Begin		End		Duration	
Begin		End		Duration	
Begin		End		Duration	

Location

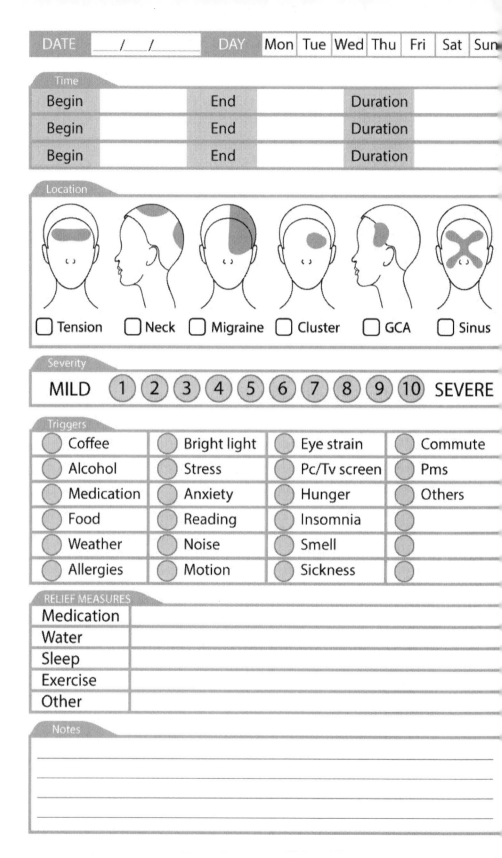

- ☐ Tension
- ☐ Neck
- ☐ Migraine
- ☐ Cluster
- ☐ GCA
- ☐ Sinus

Severity

MILD (1) (2) (3) (4) (5) (6) (7) (8) (9) (10) SEVERE

Triggers

◯ Coffee	◯ Bright light	◯ Eye strain	◯ Commute
◯ Alcohol	◯ Stress	◯ Pc/Tv screen	◯ Pms
◯ Medication	◯ Anxiety	◯ Hunger	◯ Others
◯ Food	◯ Reading	◯ Insomnia	◯
◯ Weather	◯ Noise	◯ Smell	◯
◯ Allergies	◯ Motion	◯ Sickness	◯

RELIEF MEASURES

Medication	
Water	
Sleep	
Exercise	
Other	

Notes

DATE	/ /	DAY	Mon	Tue	Wed	Thu	Fri	Sat	Sun

Time

Begin		End		Duration	
Begin		End		Duration	
Begin		End		Duration	

Location

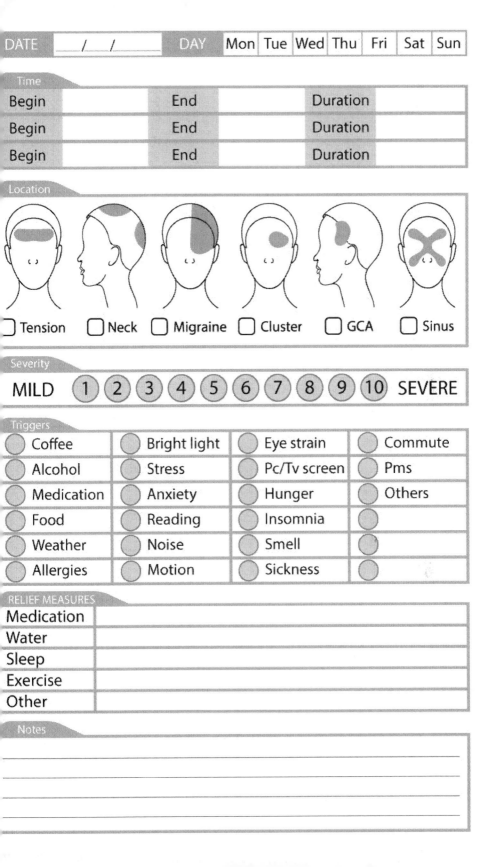

☐ Tension   ☐ Neck   ☐ Migraine   ☐ Cluster   ☐ GCA   ☐ Sinus

Severity

MILD ① ② ③ ④ ⑤ ⑥ ⑦ ⑧ ⑨ ⑩ SEVERE

Triggers

Coffee	Bright light	Eye strain	Commute
Alcohol	Stress	Pc/Tv screen	Pms
Medication	Anxiety	Hunger	Others
Food	Reading	Insomnia	
Weather	Noise	Smell	
Allergies	Motion	Sickness	

RELIEF MEASURES

Medication	
Water	
Sleep	
Exercise	
Other	

Notes

| DATE | / / | DAY | Mon | Tue | Wed | Thu | Fri | Sat | Sun |

Time

Begin		End		Duration	
Begin		End		Duration	
Begin		End		Duration	

Location

- ☐ Tension
- ☐ Neck
- ☐ Migraine
- ☐ Cluster
- ☐ GCA
- ☐ Sinus

Severity

MILD ① ② ③ ④ ⑤ ⑥ ⑦ ⑧ ⑨ ⑩ SEVERE

Triggers

◯ Coffee	◯ Bright light	◯ Eye strain	◯ Commute
◯ Alcohol	◯ Stress	◯ Pc/Tv screen	◯ Pms
◯ Medication	◯ Anxiety	◯ Hunger	◯ Others
◯ Food	◯ Reading	◯ Insomnia	◯
◯ Weather	◯ Noise	◯ Smell	◯
◯ Allergies	◯ Motion	◯ Sickness	◯

RELIEF MEASURES

Medication	
Water	
Sleep	
Exercise	
Other	

Notes

DATE	_____/_____/_____	DAY	Mon	Tue	Wed	Thu	Fri	Sat	Sun

Time

Begin		End		Duration	
Begin		End		Duration	
Begin		End		Duration	

Location

☐ Tension ☐ Neck ☐ Migraine ☐ Cluster ☐ GCA ☐ Sinus

Severity

MILD ① ② ③ ④ ⑤ ⑥ ⑦ ⑧ ⑨ ⑩ SEVERE

Triggers

◯ Coffee	◯ Bright light	◯ Eye strain	◯ Commute
◯ Alcohol	◯ Stress	◯ Pc/Tv screen	◯ Pms
◯ Medication	◯ Anxiety	◯ Hunger	◯ Others
◯ Food	◯ Reading	◯ Insomnia	◯
◯ Weather	◯ Noise	◯ Smell	◯
◯ Allergies	◯ Motion	◯ Sickness	◯

RELIEF MEASURES

Medication	
Water	
Sleep	
Exercise	
Other	

Notes

_____
_____
_____
_____

DATE	___/___/___	DAY	Mon	Tue	Wed	Thu	Fri	Sat	Sun

Time

Begin		End		Duration	
Begin		End		Duration	
Begin		End		Duration	

Location

- ☐ Tension
- ☐ Neck
- ☐ Migraine
- ☐ Cluster
- ☐ GCA
- ☐ Sinus

Severity

MILD ① ② ③ ④ ⑤ ⑥ ⑦ ⑧ ⑨ ⑩ SEVERE

Triggers

○ Coffee	○ Bright light	○ Eye strain	○ Commute
○ Alcohol	○ Stress	○ Pc/Tv screen	○ Pms
○ Medication	○ Anxiety	○ Hunger	○ Others
○ Food	○ Reading	○ Insomnia	○
○ Weather	○ Noise	○ Smell	○
○ Allergies	○ Motion	○ Sickness	○

RELIEF MEASURES

Medication	
Water	
Sleep	
Exercise	
Other	

Notes

DATE	/ /	DAY	Mon	Tue	Wed	Thu	Fri	Sat	Sun

Time

Begin		End		Duration	
Begin		End		Duration	
Begin		End		Duration	

Location

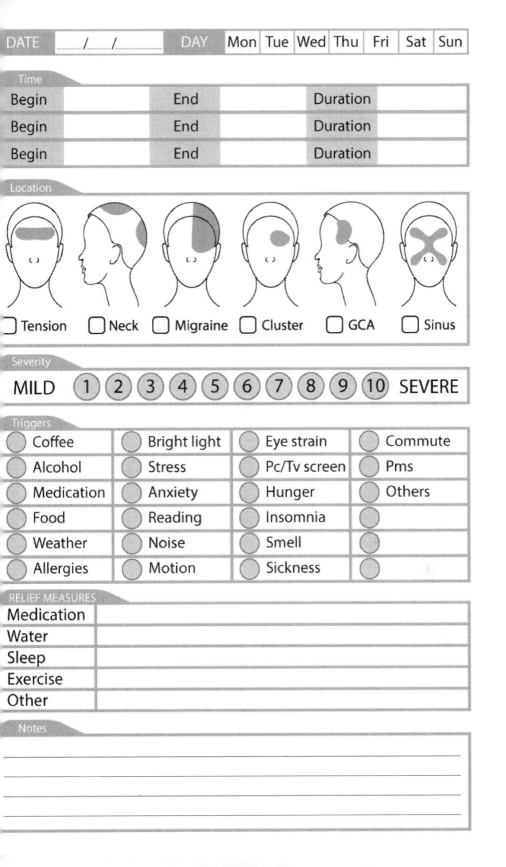

☐ Tension ☐ Neck ☐ Migraine ☐ Cluster ☐ GCA ☐ Sinus

Severity

MILD (1) (2) (3) (4) (5) (6) (7) (8) (9) (10) SEVERE

Triggers

Coffee	Bright light	Eye strain	Commute
Alcohol	Stress	Pc/Tv screen	Pms
Medication	Anxiety	Hunger	Others
Food	Reading	Insomnia	
Weather	Noise	Smell	
Allergies	Motion	Sickness	

RELIEF MEASURES

Medication	
Water	
Sleep	
Exercise	
Other	

Notes

_____
_____
_____
_____
_____

| DATE | ___/___/___ | DAY | Mon | Tue | Wed | Thu | Fri | Sat | Sun |

Time

Begin		End		Duration	
Begin		End		Duration	
Begin		End		Duration	

Location

☐ Tension ☐ Neck ☐ Migraine ☐ Cluster ☐ GCA ☐ Sinus

Severity

MILD ① ② ③ ④ ⑤ ⑥ ⑦ ⑧ ⑨ ⑩ SEVERE

Triggers

○ Coffee	○ Bright light	○ Eye strain	○ Commute
○ Alcohol	○ Stress	○ Pc/Tv screen	○ Pms
○ Medication	○ Anxiety	○ Hunger	○ Others
○ Food	○ Reading	○ Insomnia	○
○ Weather	○ Noise	○ Smell	○
○ Allergies	○ Motion	○ Sickness	○

RELIEF MEASURES

Medication	
Water	
Sleep	
Exercise	
Other	

Notes

DATE	/ /	DAY	Mon	Tue	Wed	Thu	Fri	Sat	Sun

Time

Begin		End		Duration	
Begin		End		Duration	
Begin		End		Duration	

Location

☐ Tension ☐ Neck ☐ Migraine ☐ Cluster ☐ GCA ☐ Sinus

Severity

MILD ① ② ③ ④ ⑤ ⑥ ⑦ ⑧ ⑨ ⑩ SEVERE

Triggers

○ Coffee	○ Bright light	○ Eye strain	○ Commute
○ Alcohol	○ Stress	○ Pc/Tv screen	○ Pms
○ Medication	○ Anxiety	○ Hunger	○ Others
○ Food	○ Reading	○ Insomnia	○
○ Weather	○ Noise	○ Smell	○
○ Allergies	○ Motion	○ Sickness	○

RELIEF MEASURES

Medication	
Water	
Sleep	
Exercise	
Other	

Notes

_____
_____
_____
_____
_____

DATE	/ /	DAY	Mon	Tue	Wed	Thu	Fri	Sat	Sun

Time

Begin		End		Duration	
Begin		End		Duration	
Begin		End		Duration	

Location

☐ Tension   ☐ Neck   ☐ Migraine   ☐ Cluster   ☐ GCA   ☐ Sinus

Severity

MILD ① ② ③ ④ ⑤ ⑥ ⑦ ⑧ ⑨ ⑩ SEVERE

Triggers

◯ Coffee	◯ Bright light	◯ Eye strain	◯ Commute
◯ Alcohol	◯ Stress	◯ Pc/Tv screen	◯ Pms
◯ Medication	◯ Anxiety	◯ Hunger	◯ Others
◯ Food	◯ Reading	◯ Insomnia	◯
◯ Weather	◯ Noise	◯ Smell	◯
◯ Allergies	◯ Motion	◯ Sickness	◯

RELIEF MEASURES

Medication	
Water	
Sleep	
Exercise	
Other	

Notes

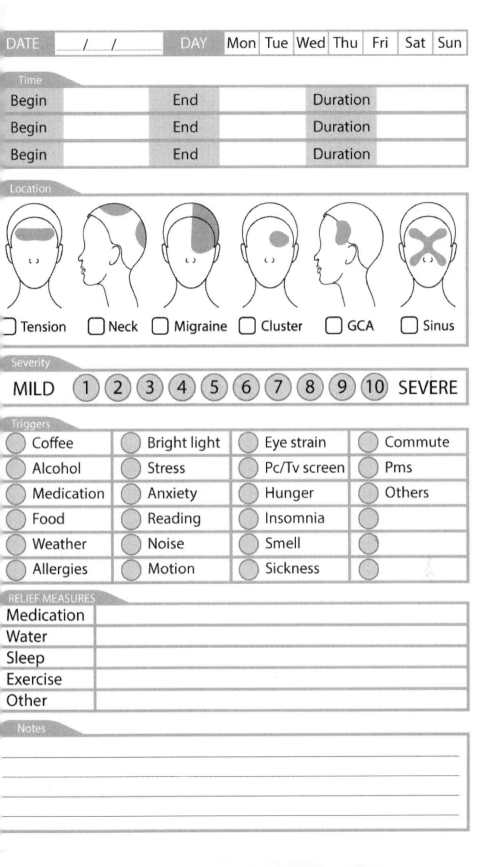

| DATE | / / | DAY | Mon | Tue | Wed | Thu | Fri | Sat | Sun |

Time

Begin		End		Duration	
Begin		End		Duration	
Begin		End		Duration	

Location

☐ Tension   ☐ Neck   ☐ Migraine   ☐ Cluster   ☐ GCA   ☐ Sinus

Severity

MILD ① ② ③ ④ ⑤ ⑥ ⑦ ⑧ ⑨ ⑩ SEVERE

Triggers

○ Coffee	○ Bright light	○ Eye strain	○ Commute
○ Alcohol	○ Stress	○ Pc/Tv screen	○ Pms
○ Medication	○ Anxiety	○ Hunger	○ Others
○ Food	○ Reading	○ Insomnia	○
○ Weather	○ Noise	○ Smell	○
○ Allergies	○ Motion	○ Sickness	○

RELIEF MEASURES

Medication	
Water	
Sleep	
Exercise	
Other	

Notes

DATE	/ /	DAY	Mon	Tue	Wed	Thu	Fri	Sat	Sun

Time

Begin		End		Duration	
Begin		End		Duration	
Begin		End		Duration	

Location

☐ Tension ☐ Neck ☐ Migraine ☐ Cluster ☐ GCA ☐ Sinus

Severity

MILD ① ② ③ ④ ⑤ ⑥ ⑦ ⑧ ⑨ ⑩ SEVERE

Triggers

◯ Coffee	◯ Bright light	◯ Eye strain	◯ Commute
◯ Alcohol	◯ Stress	◯ Pc/Tv screen	◯ Pms
◯ Medication	◯ Anxiety	◯ Hunger	◯ Others
◯ Food	◯ Reading	◯ Insomnia	◯
◯ Weather	◯ Noise	◯ Smell	◯
◯ Allergies	◯ Motion	◯ Sickness	◯

RELIEF MEASURES

Medication	
Water	
Sleep	
Exercise	
Other	

Notes

DATE	/ /	DAY	Mon	Tue	Wed	Thu	Fri	Sat	Sun

Time

Begin		End		Duration	
Begin		End		Duration	
Begin		End		Duration	

Location

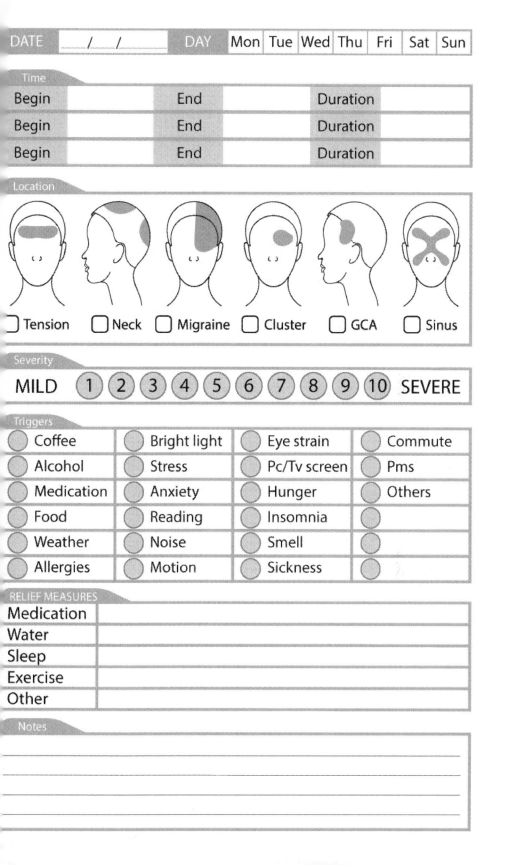

☐ Tension ☐ Neck ☐ Migraine ☐ Cluster ☐ GCA ☐ Sinus

Severity

MILD ① ② ③ ④ ⑤ ⑥ ⑦ ⑧ ⑨ ⑩ SEVERE

Triggers

○ Coffee	○ Bright light	○ Eye strain	○ Commute
○ Alcohol	○ Stress	○ Pc/Tv screen	○ Pms
○ Medication	○ Anxiety	○ Hunger	○ Others
○ Food	○ Reading	○ Insomnia	○
○ Weather	○ Noise	○ Smell	○
○ Allergies	○ Motion	○ Sickness	○

RELIEF MEASURES

Medication	
Water	
Sleep	
Exercise	
Other	

Notes

DATE	/ /	DAY	Mon	Tue	Wed	Thu	Fri	Sat	Sun

Time

Begin		End		Duration	
Begin		End		Duration	
Begin		End		Duration	

Location

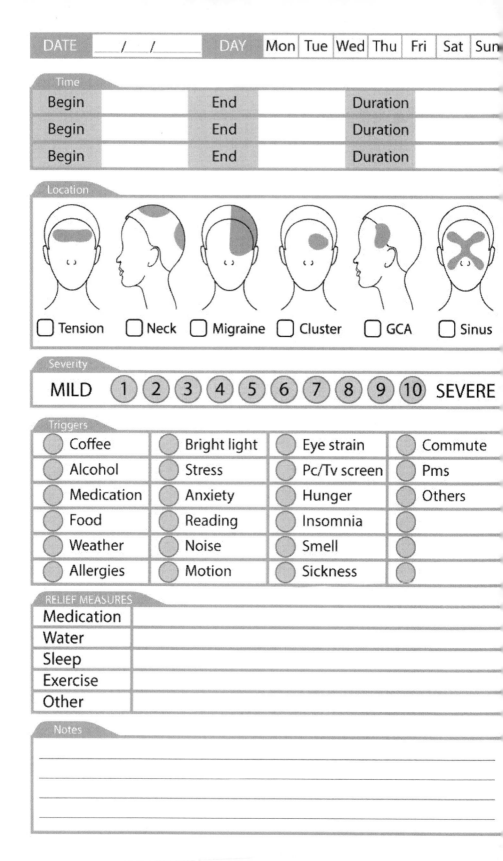

☐ Tension ☐ Neck ☐ Migraine ☐ Cluster ☐ GCA ☐ Sinus

Severity

MILD ① ② ③ ④ ⑤ ⑥ ⑦ ⑧ ⑨ ⑩ SEVERE

Triggers

◯ Coffee	◯ Bright light	◯ Eye strain	◯ Commute
◯ Alcohol	◯ Stress	◯ Pc/Tv screen	◯ Pms
◯ Medication	◯ Anxiety	◯ Hunger	◯ Others
◯ Food	◯ Reading	◯ Insomnia	◯
◯ Weather	◯ Noise	◯ Smell	◯
◯ Allergies	◯ Motion	◯ Sickness	◯

RELIEF MEASURES

Medication	
Water	
Sleep	
Exercise	
Other	

Notes

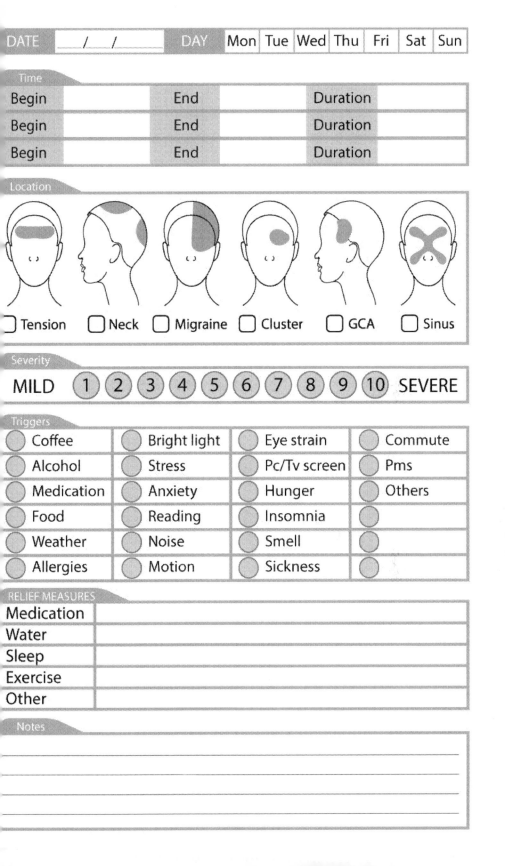

| DATE | / / | | DAY | Mon | Tue | Wed | Thu | Fri | Sat | Sun |

Time

Begin		End		Duration	
Begin		End		Duration	
Begin		End		Duration	

Location

☐ Tension ☐ Neck ☐ Migraine ☐ Cluster ☐ GCA ☐ Sinus

Severity

MILD ① ② ③ ④ ⑤ ⑥ ⑦ ⑧ ⑨ ⑩ SEVERE

Triggers

◯ Coffee	◯ Bright light	◯ Eye strain	◯ Commute
◯ Alcohol	◯ Stress	◯ Pc/Tv screen	◯ Pms
◯ Medication	◯ Anxiety	◯ Hunger	◯ Others
◯ Food	◯ Reading	◯ Insomnia	◯
◯ Weather	◯ Noise	◯ Smell	◯
◯ Allergies	◯ Motion	◯ Sickness	◯

RELIEF MEASURES

Medication	
Water	
Sleep	
Exercise	
Other	

Notes

DATE	___/___/___	DAY	Mon	Tue	Wed	Thu	Fri	Sat	Sun

Time

Begin		End		Duration	
Begin		End		Duration	
Begin		End		Duration	

Location

- ☐ Tension
- ☐ Neck
- ☐ Migraine
- ☐ Cluster
- ☐ GCA
- ☐ Sinus

Severity

MILD ① ② ③ ④ ⑤ ⑥ ⑦ ⑧ ⑨ ⑩ SEVERE

Triggers

◯ Coffee	◯ Bright light	◯ Eye strain	◯ Commute
◯ Alcohol	◯ Stress	◯ Pc/Tv screen	◯ Pms
◯ Medication	◯ Anxiety	◯ Hunger	◯ Others
◯ Food	◯ Reading	◯ Insomnia	◯
◯ Weather	◯ Noise	◯ Smell	◯
◯ Allergies	◯ Motion	◯ Sickness	◯

RELIEF MEASURES

Medication	
Water	
Sleep	
Exercise	
Other	

Notes

_____
_____
_____
_____
_____

DATE	___/___/___		DAY	Mon	Tue	Wed	Thu	Fri	Sat	Sun

Time

Begin		End		Duration	
Begin		End		Duration	
Begin		End		Duration	

Location

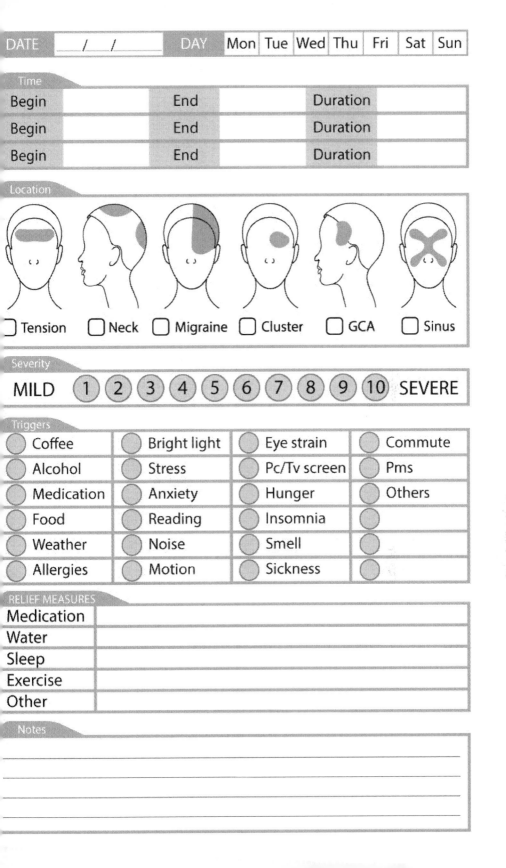

☐ Tension   ☐ Neck   ☐ Migraine   ☐ Cluster   ☐ GCA   ☐ Sinus

Severity

MILD ① ② ③ ④ ⑤ ⑥ ⑦ ⑧ ⑨ ⑩ SEVERE

Triggers

◯ Coffee	◯ Bright light	◯ Eye strain	◯ Commute
◯ Alcohol	◯ Stress	◯ Pc/Tv screen	◯ Pms
◯ Medication	◯ Anxiety	◯ Hunger	◯ Others
◯ Food	◯ Reading	◯ Insomnia	◯
◯ Weather	◯ Noise	◯ Smell	◯
◯ Allergies	◯ Motion	◯ Sickness	◯

RELIEF MEASURES

Medication	
Water	
Sleep	
Exercise	
Other	

Notes

_____
_____
_____
_____
_____

| DATE | / / | | DAY | Mon | Tue | Wed | Thu | Fri | Sat | Sun |

Time

Begin		End		Duration	
Begin		End		Duration	
Begin		End		Duration	

Location

☐ Tension   ☐ Neck   ☐ Migraine   ☐ Cluster   ☐ GCA   ☐ Sinus

Severity

MILD ① ② ③ ④ ⑤ ⑥ ⑦ ⑧ ⑨ ⑩ SEVERE

Triggers

◯ Coffee	◯ Bright light	◯ Eye strain	◯ Commute
◯ Alcohol	◯ Stress	◯ Pc/Tv screen	◯ Pms
◯ Medication	◯ Anxiety	◯ Hunger	◯ Others
◯ Food	◯ Reading	◯ Insomnia	◯
◯ Weather	◯ Noise	◯ Smell	◯
◯ Allergies	◯ Motion	◯ Sickness	◯

RELIEF MEASURES

Medication	
Water	
Sleep	
Exercise	
Other	

Notes

_____
_____
_____
_____

DATE	___/___/___	DAY	Mon	Tue	Wed	Thu	Fri	Sat	Sun

Time

Begin		End		Duration	
Begin		End		Duration	
Begin		End		Duration	

Location

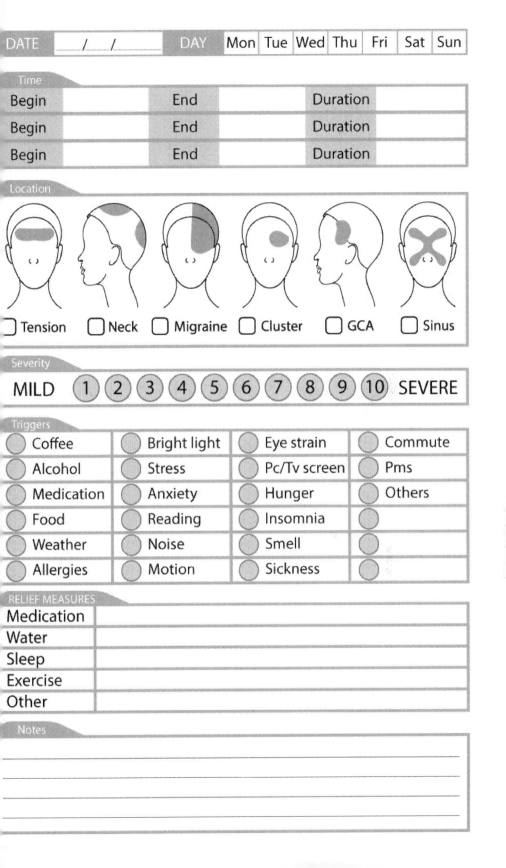

☐ Tension ☐ Neck ☐ Migraine ☐ Cluster ☐ GCA ☐ Sinus

Severity

MILD (1) (2) (3) (4) (5) (6) (7) (8) (9) (10) SEVERE

Triggers

◯ Coffee	◯ Bright light	◯ Eye strain	◯ Commute
◯ Alcohol	◯ Stress	◯ Pc/Tv screen	◯ Pms
◯ Medication	◯ Anxiety	◯ Hunger	◯ Others
◯ Food	◯ Reading	◯ Insomnia	◯
◯ Weather	◯ Noise	◯ Smell	◯
◯ Allergies	◯ Motion	◯ Sickness	◯

RELIEF MEASURES

Medication	
Water	
Sleep	
Exercise	
Other	

Notes

| DATE | / / | DAY | Mon | Tue | Wed | Thu | Fri | Sat | Sun |

Time

Begin		End		Duration	
Begin		End		Duration	
Begin		End		Duration	

Location

☐ Tension   ☐ Neck   ☐ Migraine   ☐ Cluster   ☐ GCA   ☐ Sinus

Severity

MILD ① ② ③ ④ ⑤ ⑥ ⑦ ⑧ ⑨ ⑩ SEVERE

Triggers

○ Coffee	○ Bright light	○ Eye strain	○ Commute
○ Alcohol	○ Stress	○ Pc/Tv screen	○ Pms
○ Medication	○ Anxiety	○ Hunger	○ Others
○ Food	○ Reading	○ Insomnia	○
○ Weather	○ Noise	○ Smell	○
○ Allergies	○ Motion	○ Sickness	○

RELIEF MEASURES

Medication	
Water	
Sleep	
Exercise	
Other	

Notes

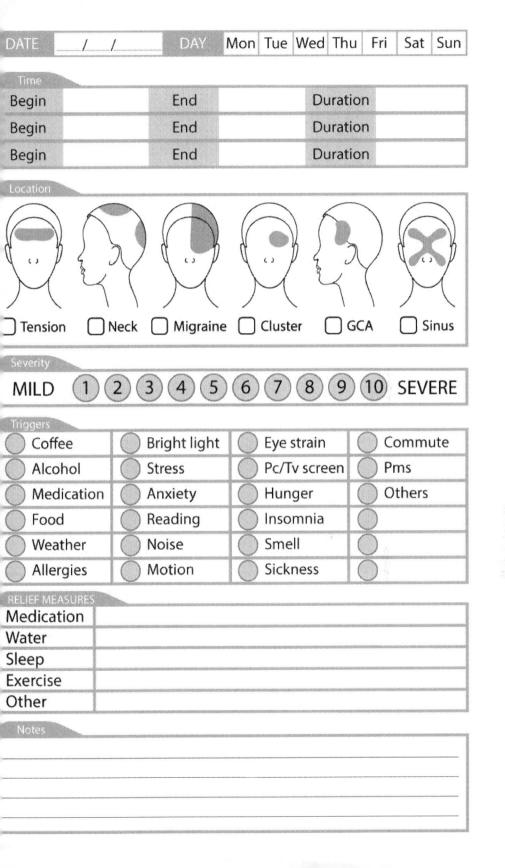

| DATE | / / | DAY | Mon | Tue | Wed | Thu | Fri | Sat | Sun |

Time

Begin		End		Duration	
Begin		End		Duration	
Begin		End		Duration	

Location

☐ Tension ☐ Neck ☐ Migraine ☐ Cluster ☐ GCA ☐ Sinus

Severity

MILD ① ② ③ ④ ⑤ ⑥ ⑦ ⑧ ⑨ ⑩ SEVERE

Triggers

◯ Coffee	◯ Bright light	◯ Eye strain	◯ Commute
◯ Alcohol	◯ Stress	◯ Pc/Tv screen	◯ Pms
◯ Medication	◯ Anxiety	◯ Hunger	◯ Others
◯ Food	◯ Reading	◯ Insomnia	◯
◯ Weather	◯ Noise	◯ Smell	◯
◯ Allergies	◯ Motion	◯ Sickness	◯

RELIEF MEASURES

Medication	
Water	
Sleep	
Exercise	
Other	

Notes

DATE	/ /	DAY	Mon	Tue	Wed	Thu	Fri	Sat	Sun

Time

Begin		End		Duration	
Begin		End		Duration	
Begin		End		Duration	

Location

☐ Tension ☐ Neck ☐ Migraine ☐ Cluster ☐ GCA ☐ Sinus

Severity

MILD ① ② ③ ④ ⑤ ⑥ ⑦ ⑧ ⑨ ⑩ SEVERE

Triggers

○ Coffee	○ Bright light	○ Eye strain	○ Commute
○ Alcohol	○ Stress	○ Pc/Tv screen	○ Pms
○ Medication	○ Anxiety	○ Hunger	○ Others
○ Food	○ Reading	○ Insomnia	○
○ Weather	○ Noise	○ Smell	○
○ Allergies	○ Motion	○ Sickness	○

RELIEF MEASURES

Medication	
Water	
Sleep	
Exercise	
Other	

Notes

DATE	/ /	DAY	Mon	Tue	Wed	Thu	Fri	Sat	Sun

Time

Begin		End		Duration	
Begin		End		Duration	
Begin		End		Duration	

Location

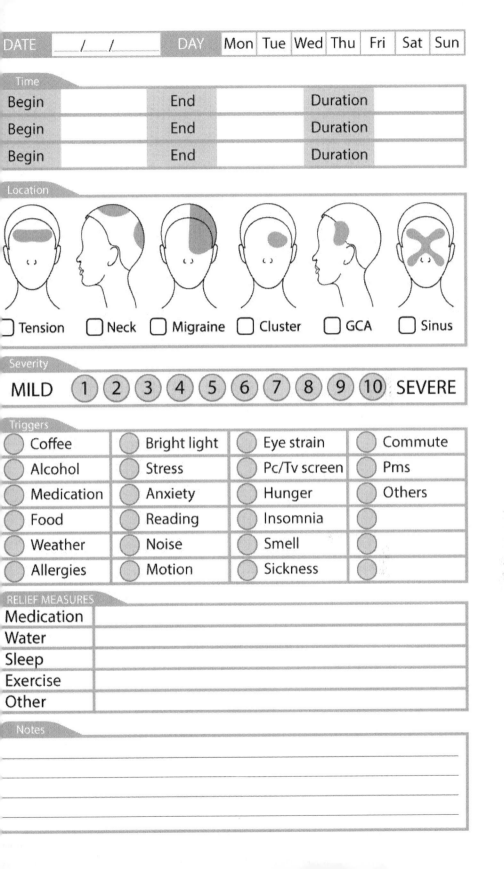

☐ Tension ☐ Neck ☐ Migraine ☐ Cluster ☐ GCA ☐ Sinus

Severity

MILD ① ② ③ ④ ⑤ ⑥ ⑦ ⑧ ⑨ ⑩ SEVERE

Triggers

◯ Coffee	◯ Bright light	◯ Eye strain	◯ Commute
◯ Alcohol	◯ Stress	◯ Pc/Tv screen	◯ Pms
◯ Medication	◯ Anxiety	◯ Hunger	◯ Others
◯ Food	◯ Reading	◯ Insomnia	◯
◯ Weather	◯ Noise	◯ Smell	◯
◯ Allergies	◯ Motion	◯ Sickness	◯

RELIEF MEASURES

Medication	
Water	
Sleep	
Exercise	
Other	

Notes

| DATE | ___/___/___ | DAY | Mon | Tue | Wed | Thu | Fri | Sat | Sun |

Time

Begin		End		Duration	
Begin		End		Duration	
Begin		End		Duration	

Location

- ☐ Tension
- ☐ Neck
- ☐ Migraine
- ☐ Cluster
- ☐ GCA
- ☐ Sinus

Severity

MILD ① ② ③ ④ ⑤ ⑥ ⑦ ⑧ ⑨ ⑩ SEVERE

Triggers

◯ Coffee	◯ Bright light	◯ Eye strain	◯ Commute
◯ Alcohol	◯ Stress	◯ Pc/Tv screen	◯ Pms
◯ Medication	◯ Anxiety	◯ Hunger	◯ Others
◯ Food	◯ Reading	◯ Insomnia	◯
◯ Weather	◯ Noise	◯ Smell	◯
◯ Allergies	◯ Motion	◯ Sickness	◯

RELIEF MEASURES

Medication	
Water	
Sleep	
Exercise	
Other	

Notes

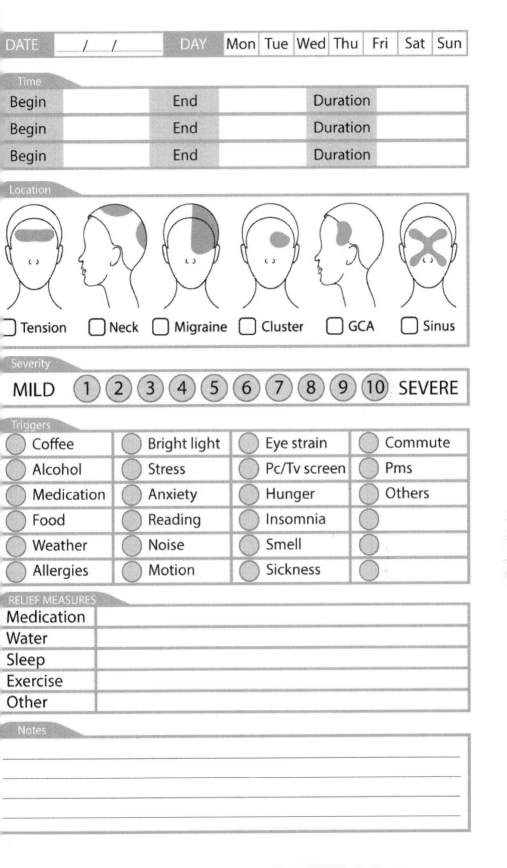

| DATE | / / | | DAY | Mon | Tue | Wed | Thu | Fri | Sat | Sun |

Time

Begin		End		Duration	
Begin		End		Duration	
Begin		End		Duration	

Location

☐ Tension ☐ Neck ☐ Migraine ☐ Cluster ☐ GCA ☐ Sinus

Severity

MILD ① ② ③ ④ ⑤ ⑥ ⑦ ⑧ ⑨ ⑩ SEVERE

Triggers

◯ Coffee	◯ Bright light	◯ Eye strain	◯ Commute
◯ Alcohol	◯ Stress	◯ Pc/Tv screen	◯ Pms
◯ Medication	◯ Anxiety	◯ Hunger	◯ Others
◯ Food	◯ Reading	◯ Insomnia	◯
◯ Weather	◯ Noise	◯ Smell	◯
◯ Allergies	◯ Motion	◯ Sickness	◯

RELIEF MEASURES

Medication	
Water	
Sleep	
Exercise	
Other	

Notes

DATE	/ /	DAY	Mon	Tue	Wed	Thu	Fri	Sat	Sun

Time

Begin		End		Duration	
Begin		End		Duration	
Begin		End		Duration	

Location

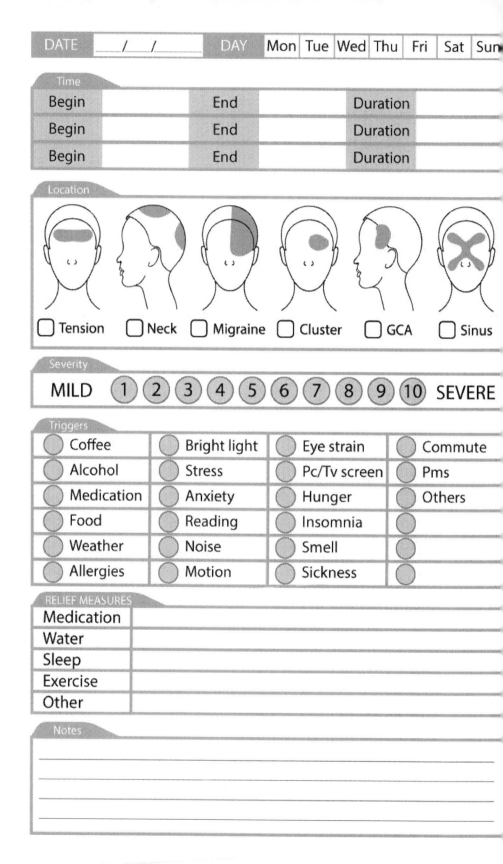

☐ Tension   ☐ Neck   ☐ Migraine   ☐ Cluster   ☐ GCA   ☐ Sinus

Severity

MILD ① ② ③ ④ ⑤ ⑥ ⑦ ⑧ ⑨ ⑩ SEVERE

Triggers

◯ Coffee	◯ Bright light	◯ Eye strain	◯ Commute
◯ Alcohol	◯ Stress	◯ Pc/Tv screen	◯ Pms
◯ Medication	◯ Anxiety	◯ Hunger	◯ Others
◯ Food	◯ Reading	◯ Insomnia	◯
◯ Weather	◯ Noise	◯ Smell	◯
◯ Allergies	◯ Motion	◯ Sickness	◯

RELIEF MEASURES

Medication	
Water	
Sleep	
Exercise	
Other	

Notes

_____
_____
_____
_____

DATE	/ /	DAY	Mon	Tue	Wed	Thu	Fri	Sat	Sun

Time

Begin		End		Duration	
Begin		End		Duration	
Begin		End		Duration	

Location

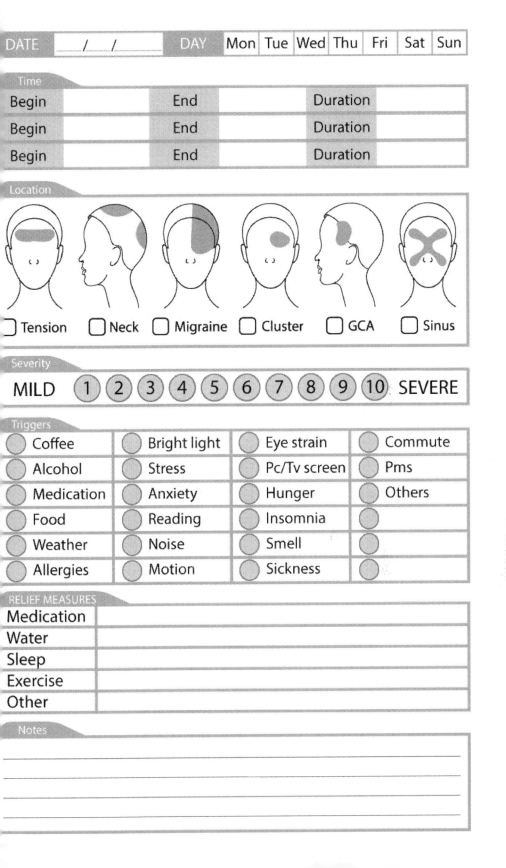

☐ Tension ☐ Neck ☐ Migraine ☐ Cluster ☐ GCA ☐ Sinus

Severity

MILD ① ② ③ ④ ⑤ ⑥ ⑦ ⑧ ⑨ ⑩ SEVERE

Triggers

○ Coffee	○ Bright light	○ Eye strain	○ Commute
○ Alcohol	○ Stress	○ Pc/Tv screen	○ Pms
○ Medication	○ Anxiety	○ Hunger	○ Others
○ Food	○ Reading	○ Insomnia	○
○ Weather	○ Noise	○ Smell	○
○ Allergies	○ Motion	○ Sickness	○

RELIEF MEASURES

Medication	
Water	
Sleep	
Exercise	
Other	

Notes

DATE	/ /	DAY	Mon	Tue	Wed	Thu	Fri	Sat	Sun

Time

Begin		End		Duration	
Begin		End		Duration	
Begin		End		Duration	

Location

☐ Tension ☐ Neck ☐ Migraine ☐ Cluster ☐ GCA ☐ Sinus

Severity

MILD ① ② ③ ④ ⑤ ⑥ ⑦ ⑧ ⑨ ⑩ SEVERE

Triggers

Coffee	Bright light	Eye strain	Commute
Alcohol	Stress	Pc/Tv screen	Pms
Medication	Anxiety	Hunger	Others
Food	Reading	Insomnia	
Weather	Noise	Smell	
Allergies	Motion	Sickness	

RELIEF MEASURES

Medication	
Water	
Sleep	
Exercise	
Other	

Notes

_____
_____
_____
_____

| DATE | / / | DAY | Mon | Tue | Wed | Thu | Fri | Sat | Sun |

Time

Begin		End		Duration	
Begin		End		Duration	
Begin		End		Duration	

Location

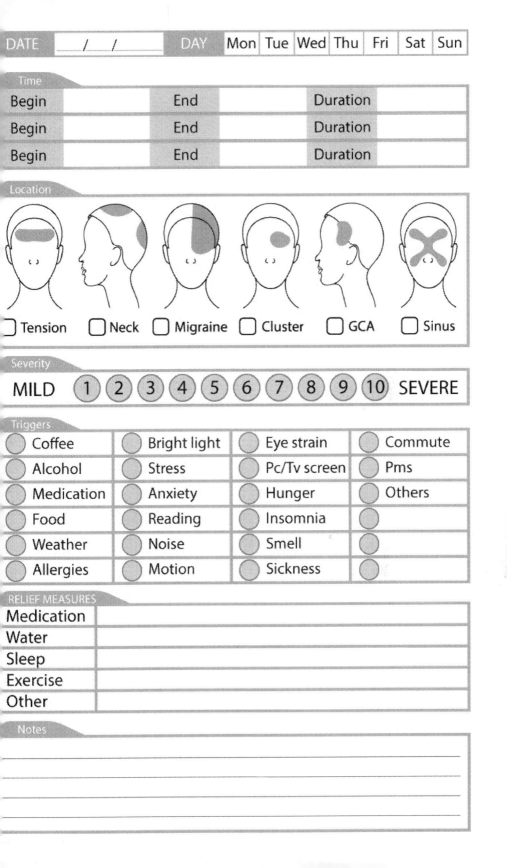

☐ Tension   ☐ Neck   ☐ Migraine   ☐ Cluster   ☐ GCA   ☐ Sinus

Severity

MILD ① ② ③ ④ ⑤ ⑥ ⑦ ⑧ ⑨ ⑩ SEVERE

Triggers

○ Coffee	○ Bright light	○ Eye strain	○ Commute
○ Alcohol	○ Stress	○ Pc/Tv screen	○ Pms
○ Medication	○ Anxiety	○ Hunger	○ Others
○ Food	○ Reading	○ Insomnia	○
○ Weather	○ Noise	○ Smell	○
○ Allergies	○ Motion	○ Sickness	○

RELIEF MEASURES

Medication	
Water	
Sleep	
Exercise	
Other	

Notes

DATE	/ /	DAY	Mon	Tue	Wed	Thu	Fri	Sat	Sun

Time

Begin		End		Duration	
Begin		End		Duration	
Begin		End		Duration	

Location

☐ Tension ☐ Neck ☐ Migraine ☐ Cluster ☐ GCA ☐ Sinus

Severity

MILD (1) (2) (3) (4) (5) (6) (7) (8) (9) (10) SEVERE

Triggers

○ Coffee	○ Bright light	○ Eye strain	○ Commute
○ Alcohol	○ Stress	○ Pc/Tv screen	○ Pms
○ Medication	○ Anxiety	○ Hunger	○ Others
○ Food	○ Reading	○ Insomnia	○
○ Weather	○ Noise	○ Smell	○
○ Allergies	○ Motion	○ Sickness	○

RELIEF MEASURES

Medication	
Water	
Sleep	
Exercise	
Other	

Notes

_____
_____
_____
_____

DATE	/ /	DAY	Mon	Tue	Wed	Thu	Fri	Sat	Sun

Time

Begin		End		Duration	
Begin		End		Duration	
Begin		End		Duration	

Location

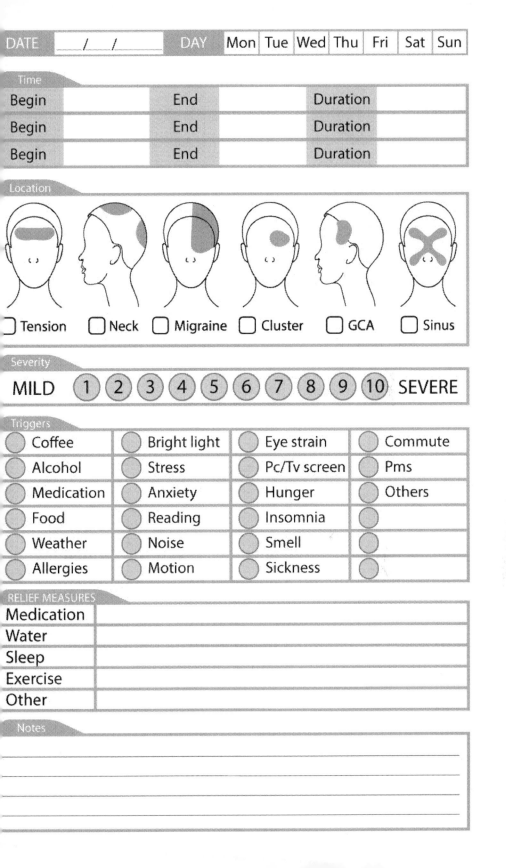

☐ Tension ☐ Neck ☐ Migraine ☐ Cluster ☐ GCA ☐ Sinus

Severity

MILD ① ② ③ ④ ⑤ ⑥ ⑦ ⑧ ⑨ ⑩ SEVERE

Triggers

◯ Coffee	◯ Bright light	◯ Eye strain	◯ Commute
◯ Alcohol	◯ Stress	◯ Pc/Tv screen	◯ Pms
◯ Medication	◯ Anxiety	◯ Hunger	◯ Others
◯ Food	◯ Reading	◯ Insomnia	◯
◯ Weather	◯ Noise	◯ Smell	◯
◯ Allergies	◯ Motion	◯ Sickness	◯

RELIEF MEASURES

Medication	
Water	
Sleep	
Exercise	
Other	

Notes

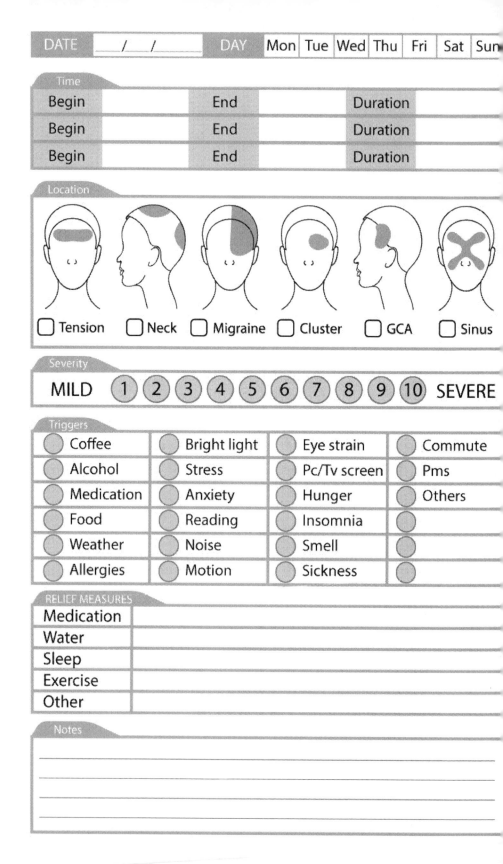

DATE	/ /	DAY	Mon	Tue	Wed	Thu	Fri	Sat	Sun

Time

Begin		End		Duration	
Begin		End		Duration	
Begin		End		Duration	

Location

☐ Tension   ☐ Neck   ☐ Migraine   ☐ Cluster   ☐ GCA   ☐ Sinus

Severity

MILD ① ② ③ ④ ⑤ ⑥ ⑦ ⑧ ⑨ ⑩ SEVERE

Triggers

○ Coffee	○ Bright light	○ Eye strain	○ Commute
○ Alcohol	○ Stress	○ Pc/Tv screen	○ Pms
○ Medication	○ Anxiety	○ Hunger	○ Others
○ Food	○ Reading	○ Insomnia	○
○ Weather	○ Noise	○ Smell	○
○ Allergies	○ Motion	○ Sickness	○

RELIEF MEASURES

Medication	
Water	
Sleep	
Exercise	
Other	

Notes

DATE ___/___/___	DAY	Mon	Tue	Wed	Thu	Fri	Sat	Sun

Time

Begin		End		Duration	
Begin		End		Duration	
Begin		End		Duration	

Location

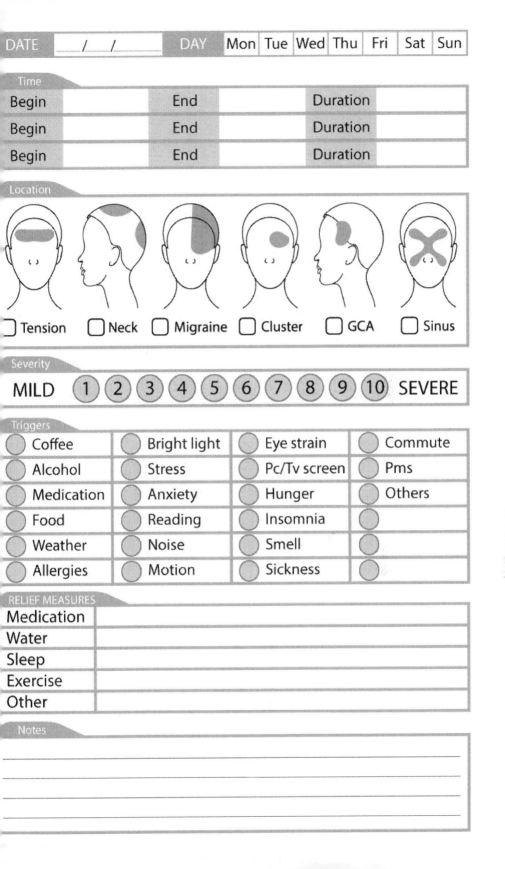

☐ Tension   ☐ Neck   ☐ Migraine   ☐ Cluster   ☐ GCA   ☐ Sinus

Severity

MILD (1) (2) (3) (4) (5) (6) (7) (8) (9) (10) SEVERE

Triggers

○ Coffee	○ Bright light	○ Eye strain	○ Commute
○ Alcohol	○ Stress	○ Pc/Tv screen	○ Pms
○ Medication	○ Anxiety	○ Hunger	○ Others
○ Food	○ Reading	○ Insomnia	○
○ Weather	○ Noise	○ Smell	○
○ Allergies	○ Motion	○ Sickness	○

RELIEF MEASURES

Medication	
Water	
Sleep	
Exercise	
Other	

Notes

_____
_____
_____
_____

DATE	/ /	DAY	Mon	Tue	Wed	Thu	Fri	Sat	Sun

Time

Begin		End		Duration	
Begin		End		Duration	
Begin		End		Duration	

Location

☐ Tension ☐ Neck ☐ Migraine ☐ Cluster ☐ GCA ☐ Sinus

Severity

MILD ① ② ③ ④ ⑤ ⑥ ⑦ ⑧ ⑨ ⑩ SEVERE

Triggers

○ Coffee	○ Bright light	○ Eye strain	○ Commute
○ Alcohol	○ Stress	○ Pc/Tv screen	○ Pms
○ Medication	○ Anxiety	○ Hunger	○ Others
○ Food	○ Reading	○ Insomnia	○
○ Weather	○ Noise	○ Smell	○
○ Allergies	○ Motion	○ Sickness	○

RELIEF MEASURES

Medication	
Water	
Sleep	
Exercise	
Other	

Notes

DATE	/ /	DAY	Mon	Tue	Wed	Thu	Fri	Sat	Sun

Time

Begin		End		Duration	
Begin		End		Duration	
Begin		End		Duration	

Location

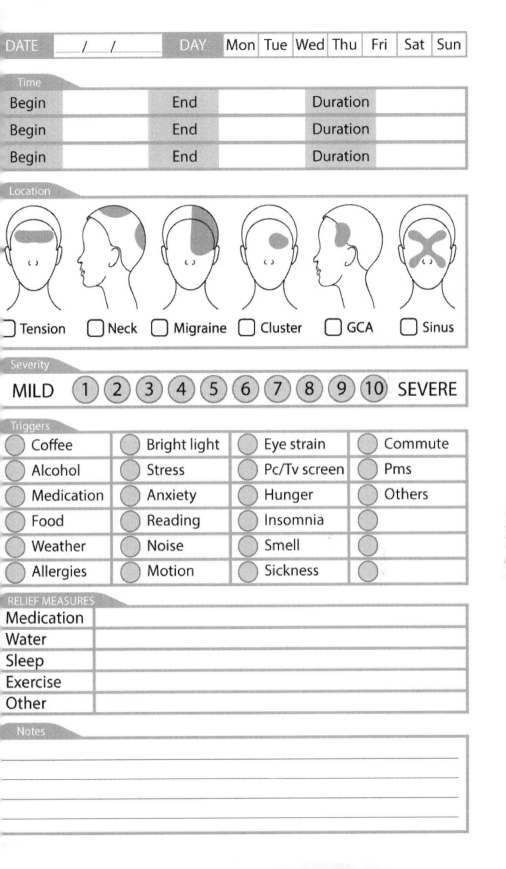

☐ Tension ☐ Neck ☐ Migraine ☐ Cluster ☐ GCA ☐ Sinus

Severity

MILD (1) (2) (3) (4) (5) (6) (7) (8) (9) (10) SEVERE

Triggers

◯ Coffee	◯ Bright light	◯ Eye strain	◯ Commute
◯ Alcohol	◯ Stress	◯ Pc/Tv screen	◯ Pms
◯ Medication	◯ Anxiety	◯ Hunger	◯ Others
◯ Food	◯ Reading	◯ Insomnia	◯
◯ Weather	◯ Noise	◯ Smell	◯
◯ Allergies	◯ Motion	◯ Sickness	◯

RELIEF MEASURES

Medication	
Water	
Sleep	
Exercise	
Other	

Notes

Time

Begin		End		Duration	
Begin		End		Duration	
Begin		End		Duration	

Location

☐ Tension ☐ Neck ☐ Migraine ☐ Cluster ☐ GCA ☐ Sinus

Severity

MILD ① ② ③ ④ ⑤ ⑥ ⑦ ⑧ ⑨ ⑩ SEVERE

Triggers

Coffee	Bright light	Eye strain	Commute
Alcohol	Stress	Pc/Tv screen	Pms
Medication	Anxiety	Hunger	Others
Food	Reading	Insomnia	
Weather	Noise	Smell	
Allergies	Motion	Sickness	

RELIEF MEASURES

Medication	
Water	
Sleep	
Exercise	
Other	

Notes

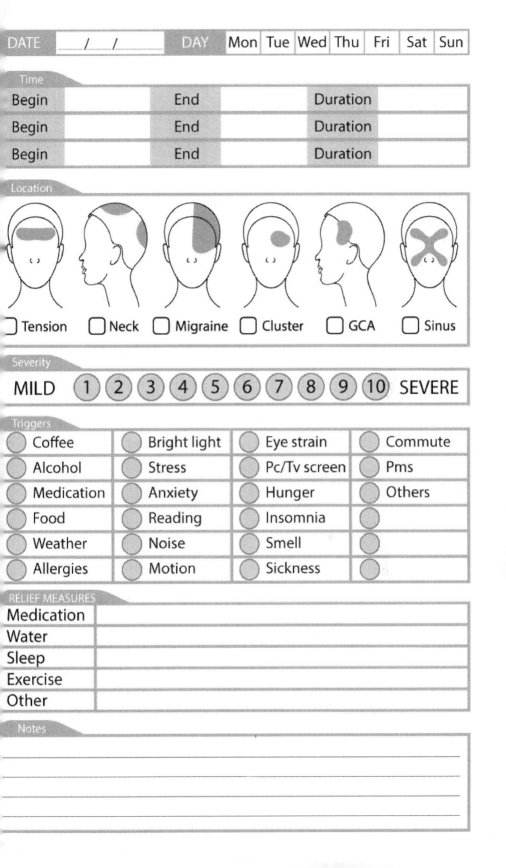

| DATE | / / | | DAY | Mon | Tue | Wed | Thu | Fri | Sat | Sun |

Time

Begin		End		Duration	
Begin		End		Duration	
Begin		End		Duration	

Location

☐ Tension ☐ Neck ☐ Migraine ☐ Cluster ☐ GCA ☐ Sinus

Severity

MILD ① ② ③ ④ ⑤ ⑥ ⑦ ⑧ ⑨ ⑩ SEVERE

Triggers

○ Coffee	○ Bright light	○ Eye strain	○ Commute
○ Alcohol	○ Stress	○ Pc/Tv screen	○ Pms
○ Medication	○ Anxiety	○ Hunger	○ Others
○ Food	○ Reading	○ Insomnia	○
○ Weather	○ Noise	○ Smell	○
○ Allergies	○ Motion	○ Sickness	○

RELIEF MEASURES

Medication	
Water	
Sleep	
Exercise	
Other	

Notes

DATE	/ /	DAY	Mon	Tue	Wed	Thu	Fri	Sat	Sun

Time

Begin		End		Duration	
Begin		End		Duration	
Begin		End		Duration	

Location

☐ Tension   ☐ Neck   ☐ Migraine   ☐ Cluster   ☐ GCA   ☐ Sinus

Severity

MILD ① ② ③ ④ ⑤ ⑥ ⑦ ⑧ ⑨ ⑩ SEVERE

Triggers

○ Coffee	○ Bright light	○ Eye strain	○ Commute
○ Alcohol	○ Stress	○ Pc/Tv screen	○ Pms
○ Medication	○ Anxiety	○ Hunger	○ Others
○ Food	○ Reading	○ Insomnia	○
○ Weather	○ Noise	○ Smell	○
○ Allergies	○ Motion	○ Sickness	○

RELIEF MEASURES

Medication	
Water	
Sleep	
Exercise	
Other	

Notes

DATE	/ /	DAY	Mon	Tue	Wed	Thu	Fri	Sat	Sun

Time

Begin		End		Duration	
Begin		End		Duration	
Begin		End		Duration	

Location

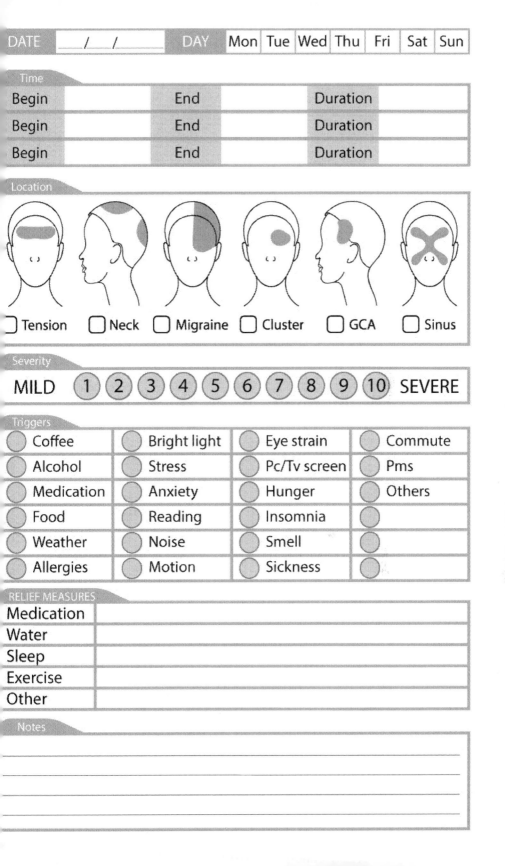

☐ Tension ☐ Neck ☐ Migraine ☐ Cluster ☐ GCA ☐ Sinus

Severity

MILD ① ② ③ ④ ⑤ ⑥ ⑦ ⑧ ⑨ ⑩ SEVERE

Triggers

○ Coffee	○ Bright light	○ Eye strain	○ Commute
○ Alcohol	○ Stress	○ Pc/Tv screen	○ Pms
○ Medication	○ Anxiety	○ Hunger	○ Others
○ Food	○ Reading	○ Insomnia	○
○ Weather	○ Noise	○ Smell	○
○ Allergies	○ Motion	○ Sickness	○

RELIEF MEASURES

Medication	
Water	
Sleep	
Exercise	
Other	

Notes

Time

Begin		End		Duration	
Begin		End		Duration	
Begin		End		Duration	

Location

☐ Tension   ☐ Neck   ☐ Migraine   ☐ Cluster   ☐ GCA   ☐ Sinus

Severity

MILD ① ② ③ ④ ⑤ ⑥ ⑦ ⑧ ⑨ ⑩ SEVERE

Triggers

○ Coffee	○ Bright light	○ Eye strain	○ Commute
○ Alcohol	○ Stress	○ Pc/Tv screen	○ Pms
○ Medication	○ Anxiety	○ Hunger	○ Others
○ Food	○ Reading	○ Insomnia	○
○ Weather	○ Noise	○ Smell	○
○ Allergies	○ Motion	○ Sickness	○

RELIEF MEASURES

Medication	
Water	
Sleep	
Exercise	
Other	

Notes

| DATE | / / | DAY | Mon | Tue | Wed | Thu | Fri | Sat | Sun |

Time

Begin		End		Duration	
Begin		End		Duration	
Begin		End		Duration	

Location

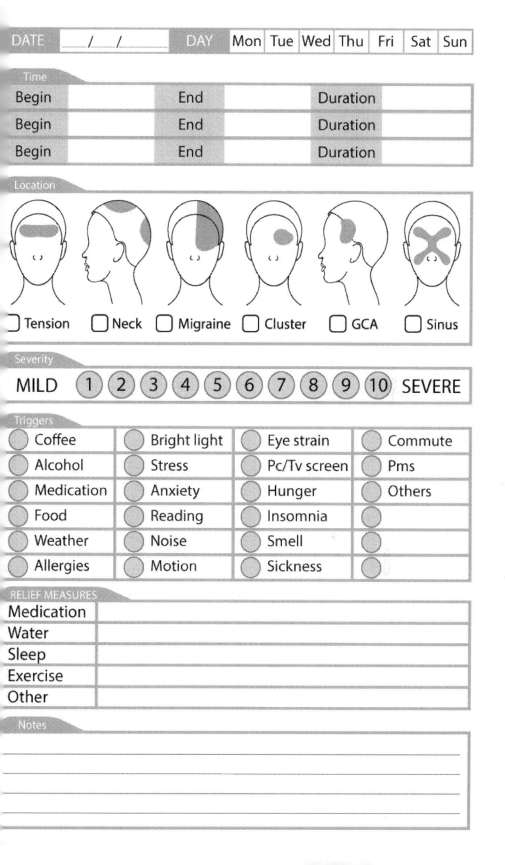

☐ Tension ☐ Neck ☐ Migraine ☐ Cluster ☐ GCA ☐ Sinus

Severity

MILD (1) (2) (3) (4) (5) (6) (7) (8) (9) (10) SEVERE

Triggers

◯ Coffee	◯ Bright light	◯ Eye strain	◯ Commute
◯ Alcohol	◯ Stress	◯ Pc/Tv screen	◯ Pms
◯ Medication	◯ Anxiety	◯ Hunger	◯ Others
◯ Food	◯ Reading	◯ Insomnia	◯
◯ Weather	◯ Noise	◯ Smell	◯
◯ Allergies	◯ Motion	◯ Sickness	◯

RELIEF MEASURES

Medication	
Water	
Sleep	
Exercise	
Other	

Notes

DATE	/ /	DAY	Mon	Tue	Wed	Thu	Fri	Sat	Sun

Time

Begin		End		Duration	
Begin		End		Duration	
Begin		End		Duration	

Location

☐ Tension ☐ Neck ☐ Migraine ☐ Cluster ☐ GCA ☐ Sinus

Severity

MILD ① ② ③ ④ ⑤ ⑥ ⑦ ⑧ ⑨ ⑩ SEVERE

Triggers

○ Coffee	○ Bright light	○ Eye strain	○ Commute
○ Alcohol	○ Stress	○ Pc/Tv screen	○ Pms
○ Medication	○ Anxiety	○ Hunger	○ Others
○ Food	○ Reading	○ Insomnia	○
○ Weather	○ Noise	○ Smell	○
○ Allergies	○ Motion	○ Sickness	○

RELIEF MEASURES

Medication	
Water	
Sleep	
Exercise	
Other	

Notes

_____
_____
_____
_____

DATE	/ /	DAY	Mon	Tue	Wed	Thu	Fri	Sat	Sun

Time

Begin		End		Duration	
Begin		End		Duration	
Begin		End		Duration	

Location

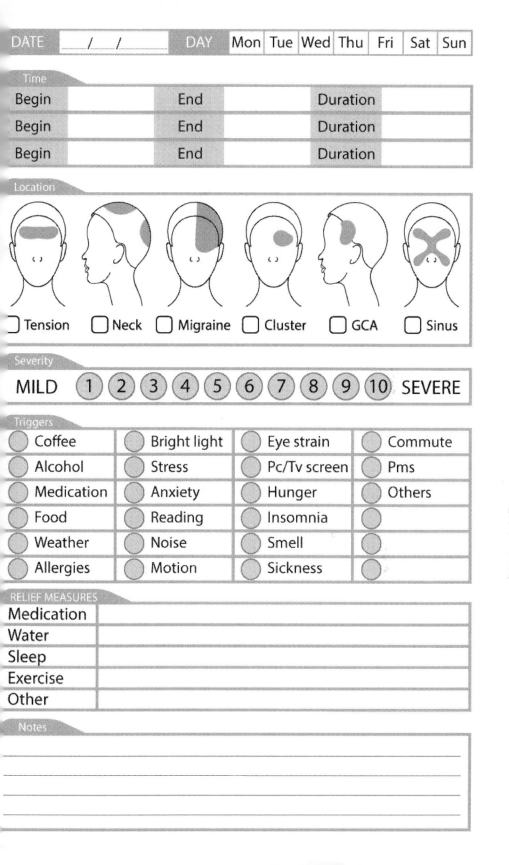

☐ Tension ☐ Neck ☐ Migraine ☐ Cluster ☐ GCA ☐ Sinus

Severity

MILD ① ② ③ ④ ⑤ ⑥ ⑦ ⑧ ⑨ ⑩ SEVERE

Triggers

○ Coffee	○ Bright light	○ Eye strain	○ Commute
○ Alcohol	○ Stress	○ Pc/Tv screen	○ Pms
○ Medication	○ Anxiety	○ Hunger	○ Others
○ Food	○ Reading	○ Insomnia	○
○ Weather	○ Noise	○ Smell	○
○ Allergies	○ Motion	○ Sickness	○

RELIEF MEASURES

Medication	
Water	
Sleep	
Exercise	
Other	

Notes

DATE	/ /		DAY	Mon	Tue	Wed	Thu	Fri	Sat	Sun

Time

Begin		End		Duration	
Begin		End		Duration	
Begin		End		Duration	

Location

☐ Tension   ☐ Neck   ☐ Migraine   ☐ Cluster   ☐ GCA   ☐ Sinus

Severity

MILD ① ② ③ ④ ⑤ ⑥ ⑦ ⑧ ⑨ ⑩ SEVERE

Triggers

Coffee	Bright light	Eye strain	Commute
Alcohol	Stress	Pc/Tv screen	Pms
Medication	Anxiety	Hunger	Others
Food	Reading	Insomnia	
Weather	Noise	Smell	
Allergies	Motion	Sickness	

RELIEF MEASURES

Medication	
Water	
Sleep	
Exercise	
Other	

Notes

DATE	/ /	DAY	Mon	Tue	Wed	Thu	Fri	Sat	Sun

Time

Begin		End		Duration	
Begin		End		Duration	
Begin		End		Duration	

Location

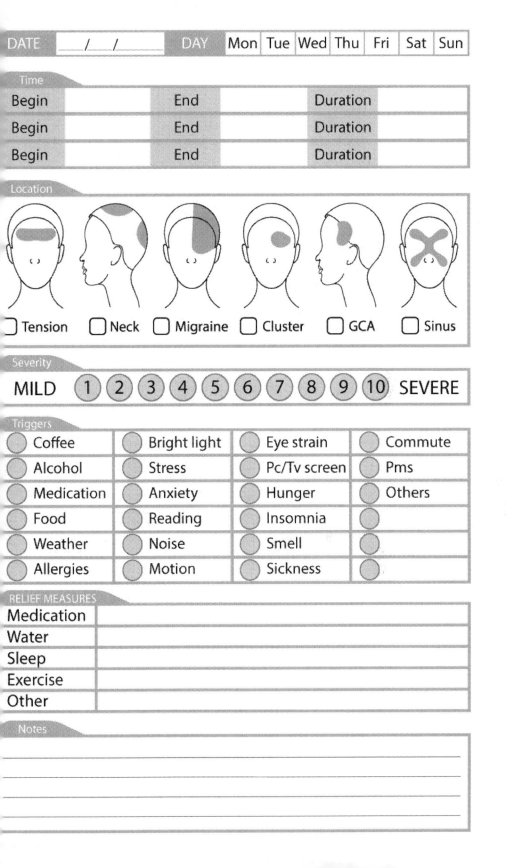

☐ Tension   ☐ Neck   ☐ Migraine   ☐ Cluster   ☐ GCA   ☐ Sinus

Severity

MILD ① ② ③ ④ ⑤ ⑥ ⑦ ⑧ ⑨ ⑩ SEVERE

Triggers

○ Coffee	○ Bright light	○ Eye strain	○ Commute
○ Alcohol	○ Stress	○ Pc/Tv screen	○ Pms
○ Medication	○ Anxiety	○ Hunger	○ Others
○ Food	○ Reading	○ Insomnia	○
○ Weather	○ Noise	○ Smell	○
○ Allergies	○ Motion	○ Sickness	○

RELIEF MEASURES

Medication	
Water	
Sleep	
Exercise	
Other	

Notes

_____
_____
_____
_____

DATE	/ /	DAY	Mon	Tue	Wed	Thu	Fri	Sat	Sun

Time

Begin		End		Duration	
Begin		End		Duration	
Begin		End		Duration	

Location

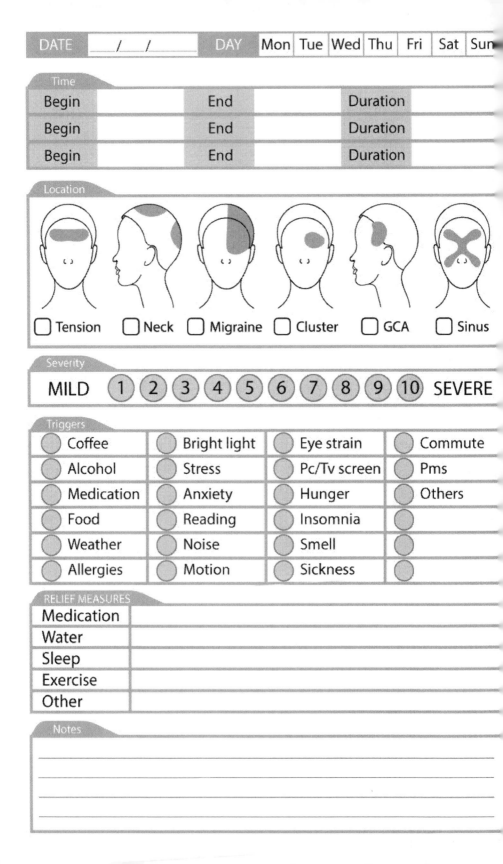

☐ Tension   ☐ Neck   ☐ Migraine   ☐ Cluster   ☐ GCA   ☐ Sinus

Severity

MILD ① ② ③ ④ ⑤ ⑥ ⑦ ⑧ ⑨ ⑩ SEVERE

Triggers

○ Coffee	○ Bright light	○ Eye strain	○ Commute
○ Alcohol	○ Stress	○ Pc/Tv screen	○ Pms
○ Medication	○ Anxiety	○ Hunger	○ Others
○ Food	○ Reading	○ Insomnia	○
○ Weather	○ Noise	○ Smell	○
○ Allergies	○ Motion	○ Sickness	○

RELIEF MEASURES

Medication	
Water	
Sleep	
Exercise	
Other	

Notes

_____
_____
_____
_____

DATE	/ /	DAY	Mon	Tue	Wed	Thu	Fri	Sat	Sun

Time

Begin		End		Duration	
Begin		End		Duration	
Begin		End		Duration	

Location

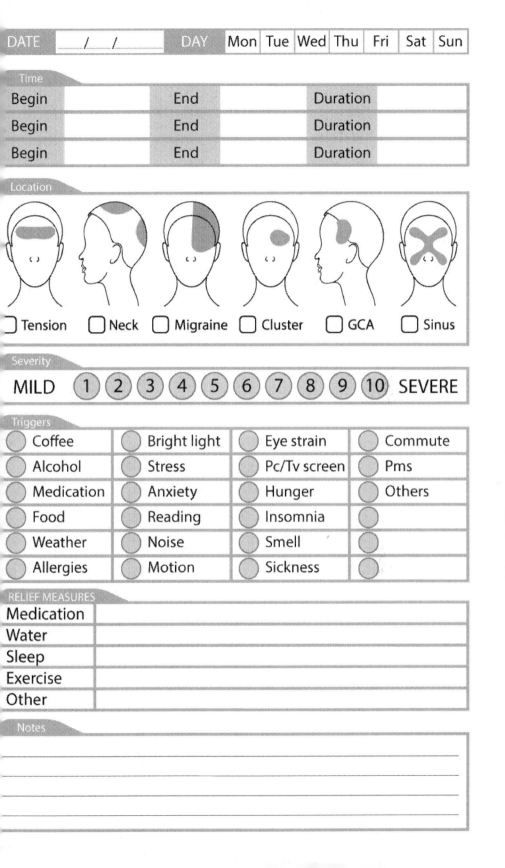

☐ Tension   ☐ Neck   ☐ Migraine   ☐ Cluster   ☐ GCA   ☐ Sinus

Severity

MILD (1) (2) (3) (4) (5) (6) (7) (8) (9) (10) SEVERE

Triggers

Coffee	Bright light	Eye strain	Commute
Alcohol	Stress	Pc/Tv screen	Pms
Medication	Anxiety	Hunger	Others
Food	Reading	Insomnia	
Weather	Noise	Smell	
Allergies	Motion	Sickness	

RELIEF MEASURES

Medication	
Water	
Sleep	
Exercise	
Other	

Notes

| DATE | / / | DAY | Mon | Tue | Wed | Thu | Fri | Sat | Sun |

Time

Begin		End		Duration	
Begin		End		Duration	
Begin		End		Duration	

Location

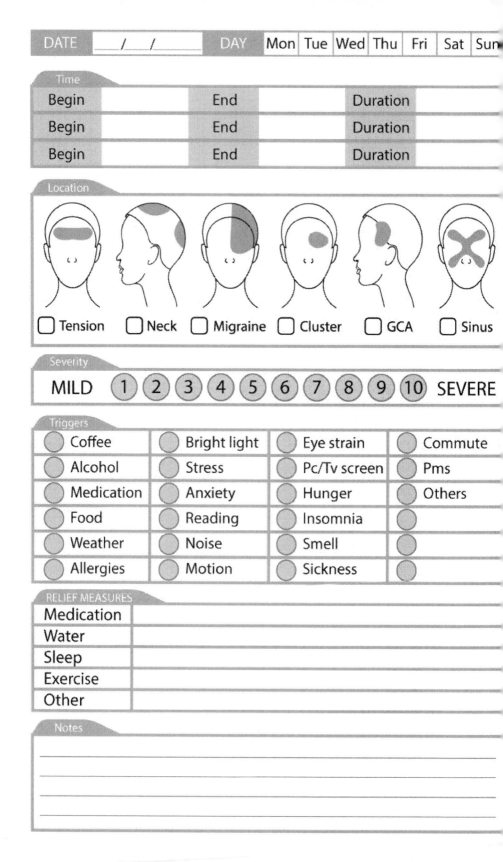

- ☐ Tension
- ☐ Neck
- ☐ Migraine
- ☐ Cluster
- ☐ GCA
- ☐ Sinus

Severity

MILD ① ② ③ ④ ⑤ ⑥ ⑦ ⑧ ⑨ ⑩ SEVERE

Triggers

◯ Coffee	◯ Bright light	◯ Eye strain	◯ Commute
◯ Alcohol	◯ Stress	◯ Pc/Tv screen	◯ Pms
◯ Medication	◯ Anxiety	◯ Hunger	◯ Others
◯ Food	◯ Reading	◯ Insomnia	◯
◯ Weather	◯ Noise	◯ Smell	◯
◯ Allergies	◯ Motion	◯ Sickness	◯

RELIEF MEASURES

Medication	
Water	
Sleep	
Exercise	
Other	

Notes

DATE	/ /	DAY	Mon	Tue	Wed	Thu	Fri	Sat	Sun

Time

Begin		End		Duration	
Begin		End		Duration	
Begin		End		Duration	

Location

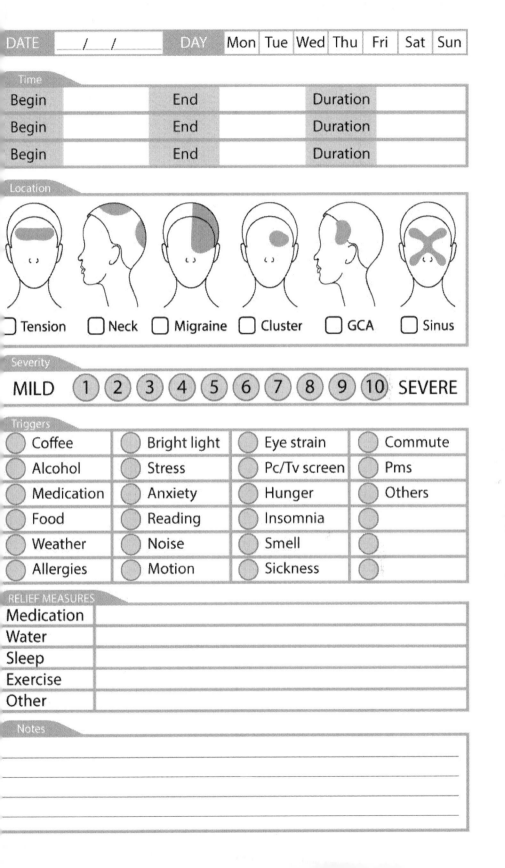

☐ Tension ☐ Neck ☐ Migraine ☐ Cluster ☐ GCA ☐ Sinus

Severity

MILD ① ② ③ ④ ⑤ ⑥ ⑦ ⑧ ⑨ ⑩ SEVERE

Triggers

○ Coffee	○ Bright light	○ Eye strain	○ Commute
○ Alcohol	○ Stress	○ Pc/Tv screen	○ Pms
○ Medication	○ Anxiety	○ Hunger	○ Others
○ Food	○ Reading	○ Insomnia	○
○ Weather	○ Noise	○ Smell	○
○ Allergies	○ Motion	○ Sickness	○

RELIEF MEASURES

Medication	
Water	
Sleep	
Exercise	
Other	

Notes

DATE	___/___/___	DAY	Mon	Tue	Wed	Thu	Fri	Sat	Sun

Time

Begin		End		Duration	
Begin		End		Duration	
Begin		End		Duration	

Location

- ☐ Tension
- ☐ Neck
- ☐ Migraine
- ☐ Cluster
- ☐ GCA
- ☐ Sinus

Severity

MILD ① ② ③ ④ ⑤ ⑥ ⑦ ⑧ ⑨ ⑩ SEVERE

Triggers

◯ Coffee	◯ Bright light	◯ Eye strain	◯ Commute
◯ Alcohol	◯ Stress	◯ Pc/Tv screen	◯ Pms
◯ Medication	◯ Anxiety	◯ Hunger	◯ Others
◯ Food	◯ Reading	◯ Insomnia	◯
◯ Weather	◯ Noise	◯ Smell	◯
◯ Allergies	◯ Motion	◯ Sickness	◯

RELIEF MEASURES

Medication	
Water	
Sleep	
Exercise	
Other	

Notes

_____
_____
_____
_____

DATE	/ /	DAY	Mon	Tue	Wed	Thu	Fri	Sat	Sun

Time

Begin		End		Duration	
Begin		End		Duration	
Begin		End		Duration	

Location

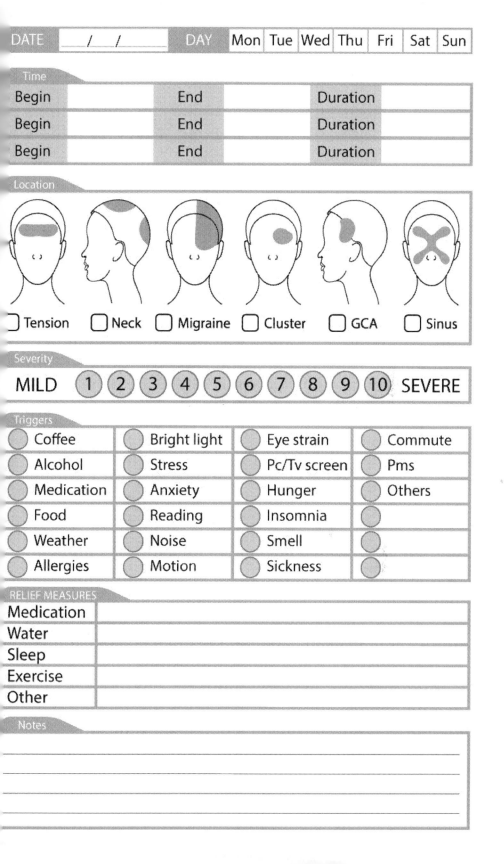

☐ Tension ☐ Neck ☐ Migraine ☐ Cluster ☐ GCA ☐ Sinus

Severity

MILD ① ② ③ ④ ⑤ ⑥ ⑦ ⑧ ⑨ ⑩ SEVERE

Triggers

○ Coffee	○ Bright light	○ Eye strain	○ Commute
○ Alcohol	○ Stress	○ Pc/Tv screen	○ Pms
○ Medication	○ Anxiety	○ Hunger	○ Others
○ Food	○ Reading	○ Insomnia	○
○ Weather	○ Noise	○ Smell	○
○ Allergies	○ Motion	○ Sickness	○

RELIEF MEASURES

Medication	
Water	
Sleep	
Exercise	
Other	

Notes

_____
_____
_____
_____
_____

DATE	/ /	DAY	Mon	Tue	Wed	Thu	Fri	Sat	Sun

Time

Begin		End		Duration	
Begin		End		Duration	
Begin		End		Duration	

Location

☐ Tension ☐ Neck ☐ Migraine ☐ Cluster ☐ GCA ☐ Sinus

Severity

MILD (1) (2) (3) (4) (5) (6) (7) (8) (9) (10) SEVERE

Triggers

○ Coffee	○ Bright light	○ Eye strain	○ Commute
○ Alcohol	○ Stress	○ Pc/Tv screen	○ Pms
○ Medication	○ Anxiety	○ Hunger	○ Others
○ Food	○ Reading	○ Insomnia	○
○ Weather	○ Noise	○ Smell	○
○ Allergies	○ Motion	○ Sickness	○

RELIEF MEASURES

Medication	
Water	
Sleep	
Exercise	
Other	

Notes

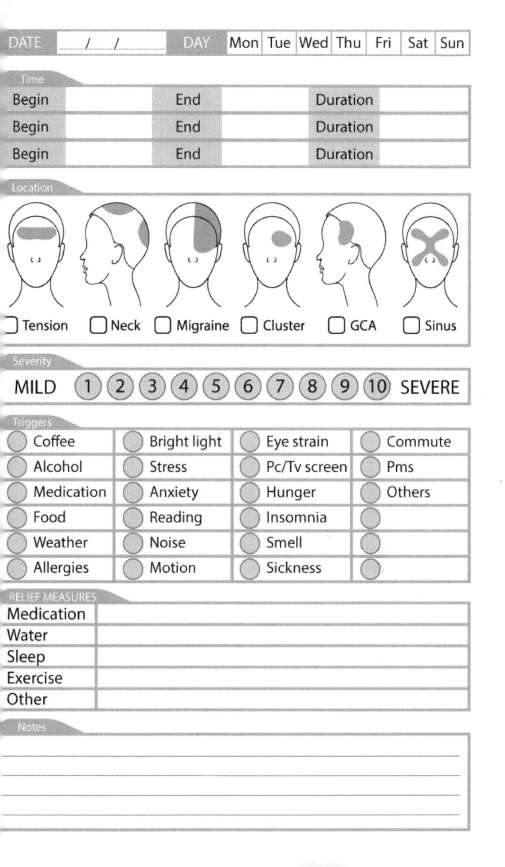

| DATE | / / | DAY | Mon | Tue | Wed | Thu | Fri | Sat | Sun |

Time

Begin		End		Duration	
Begin		End		Duration	
Begin		End		Duration	

Location

☐ Tension ☐ Neck ☐ Migraine ☐ Cluster ☐ GCA ☐ Sinus

Severity

MILD ① ② ③ ④ ⑤ ⑥ ⑦ ⑧ ⑨ ⑩ SEVERE

Triggers

◯ Coffee	◯ Bright light	◯ Eye strain	◯ Commute
◯ Alcohol	◯ Stress	◯ Pc/Tv screen	◯ Pms
◯ Medication	◯ Anxiety	◯ Hunger	◯ Others
◯ Food	◯ Reading	◯ Insomnia	◯
◯ Weather	◯ Noise	◯ Smell	◯
◯ Allergies	◯ Motion	◯ Sickness	◯

RELIEF MEASURES

Medication	
Water	
Sleep	
Exercise	
Other	

Notes

DATE	___/___/___	DAY	Mon	Tue	Wed	Thu	Fri	Sat	Sun

Time

Begin		End		Duration	
Begin		End		Duration	
Begin		End		Duration	

Location

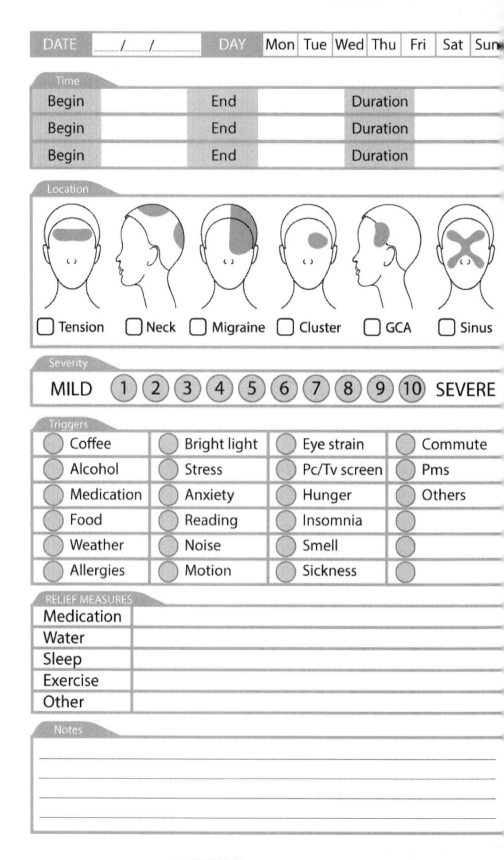

☐ Tension   ☐ Neck   ☐ Migraine   ☐ Cluster   ☐ GCA   ☐ Sinus

Severity

MILD (1) (2) (3) (4) (5) (6) (7) (8) (9) (10) SEVERE

Triggers

○ Coffee	○ Bright light	○ Eye strain	○ Commute
○ Alcohol	○ Stress	○ Pc/Tv screen	○ Pms
○ Medication	○ Anxiety	○ Hunger	○ Others
○ Food	○ Reading	○ Insomnia	○
○ Weather	○ Noise	○ Smell	○
○ Allergies	○ Motion	○ Sickness	○

RELIEF MEASURES

Medication	
Water	
Sleep	
Exercise	
Other	

Notes

DATE	/ /	DAY	Mon	Tue	Wed	Thu	Fri	Sat	Sun

Time

Begin		End		Duration	
Begin		End		Duration	
Begin		End		Duration	

Location

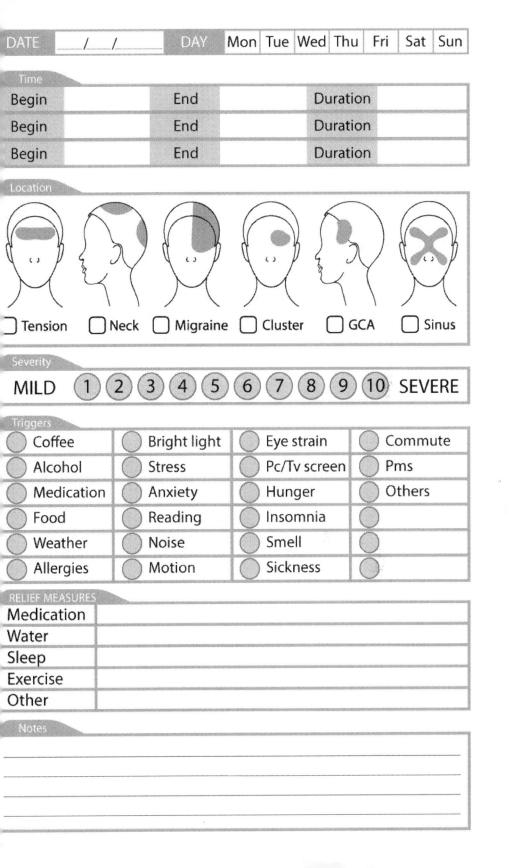

☐ Tension ☐ Neck ☐ Migraine ☐ Cluster ☐ GCA ☐ Sinus

Severity

MILD ① ② ③ ④ ⑤ ⑥ ⑦ ⑧ ⑨ ⑩ SEVERE

Triggers

○ Coffee	○ Bright light	○ Eye strain	○ Commute
○ Alcohol	○ Stress	○ Pc/Tv screen	○ Pms
○ Medication	○ Anxiety	○ Hunger	○ Others
○ Food	○ Reading	○ Insomnia	○
○ Weather	○ Noise	○ Smell	○
○ Allergies	○ Motion	○ Sickness	○

RELIEF MEASURES

Medication	
Water	
Sleep	
Exercise	
Other	

Notes

_____
_____
_____
_____

DATE	/ /	DAY	Mon	Tue	Wed	Thu	Fri	Sat	Sun

Time

Begin		End		Duration	
Begin		End		Duration	
Begin		End		Duration	

Location

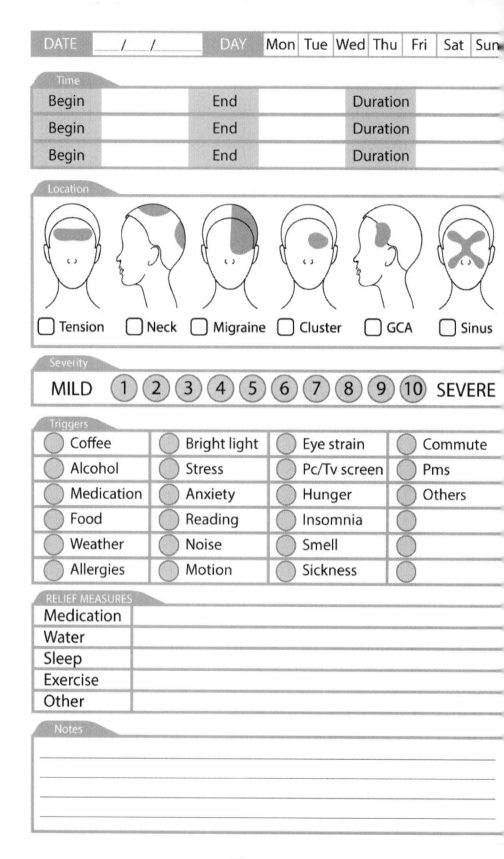

☐ Tension ☐ Neck ☐ Migraine ☐ Cluster ☐ GCA ☐ Sinus

Severity

MILD (1) (2) (3) (4) (5) (6) (7) (8) (9) (10) SEVERE

Triggers

◯ Coffee	◯ Bright light	◯ Eye strain	◯ Commute
◯ Alcohol	◯ Stress	◯ Pc/Tv screen	◯ Pms
◯ Medication	◯ Anxiety	◯ Hunger	◯ Others
◯ Food	◯ Reading	◯ Insomnia	◯
◯ Weather	◯ Noise	◯ Smell	◯
◯ Allergies	◯ Motion	◯ Sickness	◯

RELIEF MEASURES

Medication	
Water	
Sleep	
Exercise	
Other	

Notes

_____

_____

_____

_____

Made in United States
Orlando, FL
25 April 2022

17175071R00067